Advance praise for *Being Present: A Nurse's Resource for End-of-Life Communication*

"The book *Being Present* is a valuable contribution to the growing awareness that all nurses are called to care for the seriously ill and dying. It reminds us that nursing is sacred work and provides thoughtful perspectives on essential acts of being present—having difficult conversations, confronting spiritual needs, and the vital topic of nurses caring for themselves. This scholarly work is a unique resource and is rich in narratives and reflective practices for nurses."

—Betty Ferrell, PhD, MA, FAAN, FPCN
Research Scientist, Division of Nursing Research and Education
City of Hope
Duarte, California, USA

"Caring for patients at the end of life is one of the most challenging tasks in nursing practice. This is an excellent book to use in preparing nurses and nursing students to help alleviate the suffering related to death and dying. The book presents a public health perspective on dying and views the last journey as an important and healthy part of life, both for patients and their relatives. The combination of evidence from the literature, ethical knowledge, nursing stories, and questions for discussion and further reflection invites nurses into a deeper understanding of their own life, as well as providing tools to act accordingly with dying patients and their families. Reading the book with an open mind can be a transforming process for the nurse, personally as well as professionally. Using nursing stories from both the United States and Norway gives the book a cultural relevance and makes it interesting far beyond the U.S."

—Berit Sæteren, RN, PhD
Associate Professor and Head of Postgraduate Studies in Nursing
Diakonova University College
Oslo, Norway

"Medical technology provides an incredible array of tools to employ in the mission to fix and cure disease and advance the science of nursing. Schaffer and Norlander help us to understand that, perhaps, one of the most valuable tools is our ability to communicate. Their work adds to the vital discussion of how to best care for the dying patient by teaching nurses the importance of actively listening and being present to patients and their families at the end of life. In doing so, they significantly enhance the knowledge of the art of nursing."

—Kerstin McSteen, RN, MS, ACHPN
Clinical Nurse Specialist
Abbott Northwestern Hospital
Minneapolis, Minnesota, USA

"All too often, nurses and other clinicians learn the art and science of providing therapeutic interactions during the end-of-life process through complex, distressing experiences. Being truly patient- and family-centered requires coming into the caring processes as fully prepared as possible. The authors provide a framework for delivering expert compassionate care to patients and families during the end of life. The framework is action-oriented, iterative, and interactive, and it allows for the uniqueness of every patient, family, and situation. This book serves to guide clinicians at all levels—from novice to expert—in their own journey of professional identity and bolsters the strength that the clinician brings to the patient and family for end of life."

—Patricia Reid Ponte, RN, DNSc, NEA-BC, FAAN
Senior Vice President, Patient Care Services
Chief Nurse, Dana-Farber Cancer Institute
Director, Oncology Nursing and Clinical Services,
Brigham and Women's Hospital
Boston, Massachusetts, USA

Being Present

A Nurse's Resource for End-of-Life Communication

*By Marjorie Schaffer, RN, BA, MS, PhD, and
Linda Norlander, RN, BSN, MS*

Sigma Theta Tau International
Honor Society of Nursing®

Sigma Theta Tau International

Publisher: Renee Wilmeth

Acquisitions Editor: Cynthia Saver, RN, MS

Project Editor: Carla Hall

Copy Editor: C. Estelle Beaumont, RN, PhD

Proofreader: Jane Palmer

Indexer: Angie Bess, RN

Cover Design by: Gary Adair

Interior Design and Page Composition by: Rebecca Harmon

Printed in the United States of America

Printing and Binding by Edwards Brothers, Inc.

Sigma Theta Tau International

550 West North Street

Indianapolis, IN 46202

To order additional books, buy in bulk, or order for corporate use, contact Nursing Knowledge International at 888.NKI.4YOU (888.654.4968/US and Canada) or +1.317.634.8171 (outside US and Canada).

To request a review copy for course adoption, e-mail **solutions@nursingknowledge.org**, or contact Cindy Jo Everett directly at 888.NKI.4YOU (888.654.4968/US and Canada) or +1.317.917.4983 (outside US and Canada).

To request author information, or for speaker or other media requests, contact Rachael McLaughlin of the Honor Society of Nursing, Sigma Theta Tau International, at 888.634.7575 (US and Canada) or +1.317.634.8171 (outside US and Canada).

ISBN-13: 978-1-930538-82-5

Library of Congress Cataloging-in-Publication Data

Schaffer, Marjorie.
  Being present : a nurse's resource for end-of-life communication / by Marjorie Schaffer and Linda Norlander.
    p. ; cm.
  Includes bibliographical references.
  ISBN 978-1-930538-82-5
1. Terminal care. 2. Nursing. I. Norlander, Linda, 1949- II. Sigma Theta Tau International. III. Title. IV. Title: Nurse's resource for end-of-life care.
  [DNLM: 1. Nursing Care. 2. Terminal Care. 3. Nurse's Role. 4. Nurse-Patient Relations. WY 152 S525b 2009]
  RT87.T45S33 2009
  616'.029--dc22
                          2009018817

First Printing
2009

Dedication

We dedicate this book to nurses across the world who care for dying patients and their families. It is through your work that living the end of one's life has the potential to be a whole and holy experience. We hope that each of you continues to receive the strength, the rewards, and the inspiration to continue this work.

Acknowledgements

We have been inspired by our nursing colleagues who share a passion for being present with dying patients and their families. There are many who have supported us in our journey of writing this book. Lores Vlaminck reviewed our chapters as we wrote them and gave suggestions to make them better. Esther Tatley championed the Norwegian research through providing connections to the Norwegian people. The Fulbright Scholar Program made it possible for Marjorie Schaffer to travel to Norway. The Institute of Nursing and Health Sciences at the University of Oslo provided office support and supplies; the Fulbright office in Norway assisted with travel to additional geographic areas of Norway for interviews with nurses. Eli Haugen Bunch of the University of Oslo provided ideas and strategies for contacting Norwegian health professionals for interviews. Kerstin McSteen, Jody Chrastek, Kris Allen, Sue Powell, Marlaine Johnson, and Angela Lee shared their stories and insight gained from expert practice in end-of-life care. Renee Kumpula, Faith Zwirchitz, Heather Van Cleave, Laura Tierschel, and Sarah Powell are Bethel University graduate and undergraduate nursing students who have contributed to ongoing knowledge development in end-of-life nursing care through their projects and research.

Marjorie Schaffer

Linda Norlander

About the Authors

Marjorie Schaffer, RN, BA, MS, PhD

Marjorie Schaffer is a professor of nursing at Bethel University in St. Paul, Minnesota. She received her Bachelor of Science in Nursing from Gustavus Adolphus College, her master's degree from Boston College, and her PhD from the University of Minnesota. She recently completed a Fulbright Senior Scholar project, studying Norwegian nurses and their end-of-life care communication and decision-making. Schaffer is active in the Henry Street Consortium, a partnership between nursing faculty and local public health to work with nursing students and new nursing graduates on public health nursing competencies. She is also a journal reviewer for *Family Relations* and *Public Health Nursing*. Schaffer has researched and published on end-of-life decision-making, ethical issues, and public health nursing. She currently serves as president of Chi-at-Large Chapter of the Honor Society of Nursing, Sigma Theta International.

Linda Norlander, RN, BSN, MS

Linda Norlander, RN, BSN, MS, is manager of the Group Health Home Care and Hospice program in Tacoma, Washington. She is an expert on end-of life care, advance care planning, and hospice and has written and spoken extensively on these topics. She is author of *To Comfort Always: A Nurse's Guide to End of Life Care* and is co-author of *Choices at the End of Life: Finding Out What Your Parents Want Before It's Too Late* and recipient of national research grants to improve quality of care for dying patients in Minnesota. She was a Robert Wood Johnson Executive Nurse Fellow and is a member of the Honor Society of Nursing, Sigma Theta Tau International.

Table of Contents

Introduction

"I had heard about those golden moments, when the patient starts talking about something that is important or difficult to him, and you just don't listen or you don't know what to say, and later you think, 'Oh, I missed that moment.'"

Death is something most of us say we will face later. "I don't want to think about that now," we say to ourselves. Yet, for nurses who care for patients at the end of life, thinking about it *now* and talking about it *now* are critical parts of the work we do.

The reality of our work often involves concentrating on a flurry of activities and life-prolonging measures, rather than on the more difficult discussion about dying. Discussion about end of life—what is happening, what one can expect, what kinds of care are available, what is preferred—has the potential to help health care professionals, patients, and families move beyond the technological imperative to a gentler, kinder, and more natural process of dying.

This book is about opportunities and strategies for reflecting, listening, and talking with patients and families about their needs, hopes, and wishes as they face death. It is about the experiences of nurses caring for patients at the end of life. It is about how the evidence and research validate the importance of using the *golden moment* in our nursing practice. And it is a guide for using best practices as we are present with patients and families in their end-of-life journey.

Healthy Dying: A Public Health Paradigm

Both authors are public health nurses, and we think about dying from a public health perspective. A birth-to-death public health paradigm (Miller & Ryndes, 2005) indicates that effective systems, community, and individual public health strategies add healthy years to lives of individuals. But the birth-to-death paradigm also addresses the response to the dying process. Activities such as discussions with patients and families about end-of-life care can be viewed as promoting health and facilitating growth at the end of life.

We believe there are healthy ways to live and healthy ways to die. Healthy dying includes the opportunity for individuals and family members to reflect on their life experiences, contributions, regrets, meaningfulness of existence, and value of relationships.

Helping patients and families find assistance and support for good end-of-life care contributes to reduced stress, caregiver burden, and illness. Satisfaction with choices made for end-of-life health care facilitates healing of family members and helps them move forward in life. From a population health perspective, if fewer health care dollars are spent on expensive and often excessive life-saving and life-prolonging technology, additional dollars become available for other health care priorities to promote the public's health (Miller & Ryndes, 2005).

The Framework: Reflective and Ethical Practice

To learn the most and to develop greater expertise, a nurse who provides end-of-life care must be willing to embark on a reflective journey. We can view reflective practice on increasingly complex levels (Duke & Appleton, 2000).

At the first level of reflection, the nurse describes what is happening and focuses on action without thinking about the meaning of the action. In the second level of reflection, the nurse considers how nursing knowledge supports actions and opinions. The nurse makes connections and integrates the supporting knowledge, but does not necessarily change practice or examine assumptions about the correct nursing actions. In the third level, the critical/emancipatory phase (Kim, 1999), the nurse considers the bigger picture and the many factors that influence a situation. Ethical, political, spiritual, and professional issues all impact how the nurse initiates the dialogue, as well as the content of the dialogue when engaging in discussions about end of life. Nurses are also less likely to bring spiritual needs and concerns into end-of-life conversation because of concerns about privacy, a misunderstanding of the rules, a lack of knowledge of various religions, and feelings of discomfort. A nurse who has taken on the challenge of the critical/

emancipatory phase of reflective practice will examine these additional issues and consider how they impact nursing action. Once there, he or she can then move on to investigating more resources, considering alternative actions, and finally taking new perspectives that lead to changing practice. When nurses reach a level of knowing in which they consider both the best evidence for end-of-life discussion and how to engage in reflective practice, they achieve the fourth level of reflection, known as personal or deep reflection (Clarke, Kelly, & James, 1996; Duke & Appleton, 2000). At this stage, nurses both evaluate their own thinking and performance and analyze their knowledge about end-of-life care. This is in contrast to simply learning what other nurses do and acting with little reflection about reasons for their actions. Reflective practice involves mindfulness, self-awareness, consciousness and responsibility for one's actions, and a realization of one's vision (Johns, 2005). This knowledge gained from reflective practice supplies the motivation, passion, and commitment to take action in our nursing practice.

Reflective practice is enhanced by the ability to analyze and work toward resolving ethical problems. When we encounter ethical problems in caring for clients and families at the end of life, three approaches can help us understand how to respond to the conflict or tension that results from these problems:

1. rule ethics,

2. virtue ethics, and

3. feminist ethics (Volbrecht, 2002).

Most of us are very familiar with a rule ethics approach or ethical principles. From a bioethics perspective, autonomy (freedom to make decisions), justice (fairness in allocation of resources and giving people their rights), beneficence (promoting good), and nonmalificence (preventing harm) guide health care professionals in resolving a variety of ethical problems encountered in practice.

Virtue ethics expands our understanding of how we use who we are—our professional identity, our values, our beliefs about humanity—to take action when tension resulting from ethical conflict does not go away. Historically, virtue ethics developed out of Aristotle's thinking about human flourishing. Virtue ethics focuses on the development of good character within the context of living in a community. "Who should we be?" as we interact with patients, families, and other health professionals and staff is the question to answer from a virtue ethics perspective (Cameron, 2000). Many virtues help us to do good work, including compassion, courage, justice, humility, honesty, practical reasoning, resilience, and integrity.

Finally, feminist ethics helps us to consider how patients and families may experience oppression in the hierarchy of the health care system. We have inherited paternalistic inclinations stemming from a male-dominated system of the past that result in power *over*, rather than power *with* (shared power). A feminist ethics approach aims to equalize power and give voice to anyone experiencing oppression. This can be a challenge in our health care world, where inequality in importance related to gender and position still exists. From a feminist ethics perspective, nurses advocate for persons and groups whose voices are not being heard. Feminist ethics is about action—changing the status quo to a system that values everyone equally.

"I didn't realize until I started working with critically ill patients that the strongest skills I needed were not the technical skills, but rather the ability to listen to patients and families."

Rule ethics, virtue ethics, and feminist ethics—how can we keep all of these ideas in mind when responding to ethical problems, given that we have caregiving lives filled with many activities and responsibilities? Cameron (2000) developed the Value, Be, Do Ethical Decision-Making Model that helps us consider three questions as we work to understand ethical problems and how to respond to them.

1. What should I value?
2. Who should I be?
3. What should I do?

Although these three questions may seem simplistic, working through them in order helps us to determine an ethical response. First, determine the values that give meaning to your life. Then reflect on how you can live these values in your everyday actions. Behaving with integrity means that your actions are consistent with your words. Once you have reflected on your responses to the first two questions, then you can consider what resolution is consistent with your values and character. As you decide on a response (which sometimes can be no action), analyze what the right action is based on ethical principles and what the outcomes or consequences of the response might be. Also, keep in mind that we exist in a health care community, and our co-workers and interdisciplinary health care team can be of great help in working through the ethical problems we encounter.

The Nurses' Stories

The nurses' stories for this book were taken from interviews and focus groups with nurses from the United States and from Norway. The Norwegian nurses' perceptions add to our body of knowledge, because they live in a society where privacy is highly valued and protected. Under these circumstances, it takes special skills and a high degree of reflective practice to work with families at the end of life.

The nurses we worked with for this book come from a variety of settings, including hospital, hospice, home, and long-term care. They bring rich and in-depth experiences of working with patients and families dealing with dying and death. As one nurse said, "I didn't realize until I started working with critically ill patients that the strongest skills I needed were not the technical skills, but rather the ability to listen to patients and families." (personal communication)

What You Will Find in Each Chapter

It is our hope that each of the chapters will help you to think about ways to initiate and enhance communication with patients and families who are experiencing the dying process. The evidence from literature and from nurses' stories provides you with a wealth of learned wisdom that can help you create your repertoire of best practices in caring for dying patients and families. Evidence presented in this book covers a broad range of levels, including research studies on effective communication, systematic reviews of the literature, case studies, expert opinion articles, and individual stories of nurses whose everyday work is caring for dying patients and families.

Each chapter features a communication theme that is generated from nurses' stories. You will find these components in each of the following chapters:

- Best evidence for end-of-life discussion in nursing practice.

- Reflection about meaning for practice.

- Ethical practice question.

- Stories from real nurses about their experiences.

- Key points.

- Questions for discussion and further reflection.

As a nurse who mentors younger nurses explained,

> *I have learned after all these years that you have to make this golden moment, even if you don't have the time. Like the day when an elderly man said, "I can't talk to my wife. I need to speak to her about the fact I'm going to die." I was very busy, and afterwards I felt bad. When you are younger you think this moment is precious, and when it's gone you can't get it back. But this is something I try to tell the young nurses: You can go back and you can make those golden moments come back.*

We will create more golden moments of communication by learning how to be present with patients who are facing the end of life. Nurses have many things they do as they provide end-of-life care. It is in the integration of being present with our *doing* that we will make a difference for our patients and their families and improve their quality of life at the end of life.

REFLECTION QUESTIONS

1. What level of reflection do you think you are currently using in your end-of-life nursing care practice?

2. What stories come to mind as you consider your own experiences with talking to patients and families who are contemplating or experiencing the dying process?

3. What has been your experience in finding "golden moments" in conversations with dying patients and families?

References

Cameron, M. E. (2000). Value, be, do: Guidelines for resolving ethical conflict. *Journal of Nursing Law, 6*(4), 15-24.

Clarke, B., James, C., & Kelly, J. (1996). Reflective practice: Reviewing the issues and refocusing the debate. *International Journal of Nursing Studies, 33*, 167-174.

Duke, S., & Appleton, J. (2000). The use of reflection in a palliative care programme: A quantitative study of the development of reflective skills over an academic year. *Journal of Advanced Nursing, 32*(6), 1557-1568.

Johns, C. (2005). Expanding the gates of perception. In C. Johns & D. Freshwater (Eds.), *Transforming nursing through reflective practice* (pp. 1-12). Malden, MA: Blackwell Publishing.

Kim, H. S. (1999). Critical reflective inquiry for knowledge development in nursing practice. *Journal of Advanced Nursing, 29*, 1205-1212.

Miller, S. C., & Ryndes, T. (2005). Quality of life at the end of life: The public health perspective. *Generations, 29*(2), 41-47.

Volbrecht, R. M. (2002). *Nursing ethics: Communities in dialogue.* Upper Saddle River, NJ: Prentice Hall.

Additional Resources

Brown University Center for Gerontology and Health Care Research. (2001). Facts on dying: Policy relevant data on care at the end of life. Retrieved April 20, 2009, from http://www. chcr.brown.edu/dying/factsondying.htm

End-of-Life Nursing Education Consortium (ELNEC) Graduate Curriculum (2003). *Module 1: Nursing care at the end of life.* City of Hope and American Association of Colleges of Nursing.

Hamilton, J. B., III. (2001). The ethics of end of life care. In B. Poor & G. P. Poirrier (Eds.), *End of life nursing care* (pp. 73-103). Boston: Jones and Bartlett.

Kaufman, S. R. (2005). ... *And a time to die: How American hospitals shape the end of life.* New York: Scribner.

Melynk, B. M., & Fineout-Overholt, E. (2005). *Evidence-based practice in nursing and healthcare.* Philadelphia: Lippincott, Williams & Wilkins.

Rutledge, D. N., Bookbinder, M., Donaldson, N. E., & Pravikoff, D. S. (2001). End-of-life care series. Part III. Learnings beyond SUPPORT and HELP studies. *The Online Journal of Clinical Innovations, 4*(6), 1-60.

Sulmasy, D. P. (2003). Health care justice and hospice care. *Hastings Center Report* (Suppl.), S-4-S15.

White, K. R., Coyne, P. J., & Pate, U. B. (2001). Are nurses adequately prepared for end-of-life care? *Journal of Nursing Scholarship, 33*(2), 147-151.

A wife was very anxious because her husband was going to die, possibly that same evening. She had always been anxious and had cried a lot during his extended illness. I took her hand and led her into a small room. We sat down, and I said, "I have to hear how you are doing." I told her what we saw in his condition, how he could progress, and asked how she felt about being there during these final stages. I asked, "What are you frightened of? What is difficult for you?" She kept crying and finally shared with me that she was afraid of losing him and couldn't bear to see him die. I asked what she thought he would like. Would he want her there? Or would he want her crying and away from him when the end came? This was a great help to her. In fact, she genuinely wanted to be there and wanted to be calm for him. She told me later that this conversation had helped her so that she could be there.

1

•

Being Present

What does it mean to *be present* for patients and families experiencing the dying process? As nurses, we have the opportunity to comfort and guide patients and families *with* and *through* our presence. Presence is more than being physically near or at the bedside; it is a relationship with the people we are caring for. Presence is a skill and an art that can be learned and practiced.

Presence is an essential nursing intervention in care of the dying. Benner (1984) identified "presencing" as one of the eight competencies of the nurse's helping role. In a study in which patients were asked to describe experiences of feeling cared for by nurses, the researchers determined that two of eight themes were focused on the concept of presence: reassuring presence and time spent with patient (Brown, 1986). In another study, Minick (1995) found that making a connection with a patient (an aspect of presence) resulted in early identification of a problem in critically ill patients. Presence is not easily measured or quantified. However, presence can be defined, and key concepts of presence can be explored to increase understanding of how a nurse can be present in communication with dying persons and their families. As an intervention, presence is a transactional change that is viewed as meaningful by both nurse and patient (Snyder & Lindquist, 2000).

Definitions of Presence

* Being available with the wholeness of one's being (Snyder & Lindquist, 2000).

* Encountering the patient as a unique human being in a unique situation and choosing to "spend" oneself on the patient's behalf (Doona, Haggerty, & Chase, 1997).

* Intuitive knowing or sensing another's needs for help and making self physically available to be present in a helping way (Gardner, 1985).

* A subject-to-subject interrelationship that honors the ever-changing reality of the other (Parse, 1992).

Key Elements of Nursing Presence

* Attentiveness
* Accountability
* Sensitivity
* Openness
* Active Listening (Snyder, Brandt, & Tseng, 2000)

Key Elements of Nursing Presence

Being present means attending to a patient, being accountable to knowing the uniqueness of that person, developing sensitivity to the nuances of nonverbal and verbal messages, having an openness or authenticity in encounters, and being an active listener. To be present, one must know oneself and be willing to risk the vulnerability that comes with truly knowing another person.

Attentiveness

Nurses who are attentive to dying patients and their family members are "in the moment" when in the time and space of a patient and family. This means not allowing thoughts of other tasks that need to be done to crowd out thinking about the experience of that patient and family. You must choose to focus on the messages being given by the patient and family—both verbal and nonverbal. This is much more than noting the facts of the situation, physical symptoms, social history, and care strategies for patients who are dying. It is about being attentive to the patient as a unique person.

Accountability

Accountability for presence means putting one's professional power on the sidelines. It means being willing to think about what is right for patients and families from their viewpoint, rather than what is consistent with customary practice from a nursing viewpoint. Accountability also means being willing to learn from patients and families. Nurses who are accountable are intentional about investing themselves and committing the time to be present.

Sensitivity

By being present, you have the opportunity to know the patient as a unique person. This knowledge is likely to change your existing knowledge of the patient and lead to a different understanding of the situation, which ultimately contributes to better nursing judgments. These nursing judgments will be more sensitive to the patient's experience. A different understanding results from your being with the patient through the ups and downs of the changing experience often encountered in the dying process. There is no attempt to control or change the experience, the joys, or the struggles (Parse, 1992). The focus is not on tasks that may be viewed as integral to end-of-life nursing care, such as assessing the grieving process of patients and families or determining how to take away the emotional, psychological, or spiritual hurting. Rather, the focus is on what the dying patient and family members are experiencing at this moment in time. Sensitivity through presence has the potential to help patients move toward finding ways to live out hopes and dreams for the end of life (Melnechenko, 2003).

"Active listening also means working to hear the meaning behind the words."

Openness

To be present, you must be open to experiencing another person's world and open to that world. Entering another person's world requires development of one's own authentic self. This means acknowledging your own responses to death and dying, as well as areas of discomfort and not always knowing the right thing to do. This also means being open to a shared situation—both nurse and patient recognize that they are encountering a unique and significant experience. The experience of the patient and family may involve all the components of a peaceful death, or it may involve anguish and difficult relationships. Openness enhances the possibility for connection. The experience moves from a solitary experience to one of common understanding.

Nurses also need to be open to understanding their effect on others and their own self-worth, and to recognizing their own limitations (Stanley, 2000). Openness means leaving behind behaviors that result in "being distant," whether motivated by the need to be "professional" or a reaction to discomfort. An open nurse knows that people have the right to their own "becoming," and in a sense, the nurse surrenders to the situation. Being truly open is humbling (Melnechenko, 2003).

Active Listening

What is involved in active listening? Briskin described active listening as "the art of developing deeper silences in yourself, so you slow your mind's hearing to your ear's natural speed, and hear beneath the words to their meaning" (Zerwehk, 2006, p. 115).

Active listening requires engagement and quieting our own inner dialogue in order to hear our patients. This involves allowing patients to tell their stories, listening without judging or giving advice, and bearing witness to the experiences of patients (Stanley, 2002). We must remember that the stories belong to the patients and family members. Active listening also means working to hear the meaning behind the words. You will need to concentrate to pick up verbal and nonverbal cues (Edwards, 2005). This requires both attentiveness and an emotional commitment to understanding patients' stories.

Active listening often involves silence. In some situations, there may be no words of comfort that can be given. Patients may find that a nurse's physical presence and understanding of the anguish they are experiencing are more meaningful than words of comfort. When you are intentional about active listening, the outcome is unknown. You listen to hear a patient's story, rather than trying to fill in the blanks from your perspective of the patient's experience. Additional tips for active listening given by Zerwehk (2006) include the following:

- Organize the physical environment to eliminate interruptions and distractions.

- When culturally relevant, use eye contact and touch.

- Avoid questions with only yes or no answers.

- Communicate in a normal tone of voice, unless the patient is hard of hearing.

- Communicate at the same height, if possible, even if it means sitting at the bedside for a while.

- Clarify and then summarize the patient's statements to ensure you accurately understood what the patient was saying.

Empathy, Vulnerability, and Courage

Empathy may be an outcome of being present when working with dying people and their families. Martin Buber, a philosopher, integrated the concept of "inclusion" in his description of empathy. One who is empathetic steps outside of oneself and encounters the world of the other (Boston, Towers, & Barnard, 2001). However, empathy does not mean thinking or feeling like the other person. There is a sharing but also a standing apart from the other. Closeness is experienced and a bond is established, but you retain a separate identity (Travelbee, 1966). Empathy in end-of-life nursing care may bring to the nurse the insight that it is impossible to fully know the experience of the dying person (Boston et al.).

"To be empathetic, you also must be vulnerable and courageous."

To be empathetic, you also must be vulnerable and courageous. You risk emotional vulnerability when truly being present with another (Pettigrew, 1990).

It is important to clarify here the difference between sympathy and empathy. A sympathetic nurse is not present with another; rather the focus is protecting or controlling the other, expecting a specific response to one's assistance, or fixating on solutions. In contrast, the empathetic nurse focuses on feelings and relationships and can let go of the need to control the actions of another (Borne, 2001). The dying process in particular can be laden with emotional challenges. Vulnerability involves humility in being willing to be a part of the patient's learning process and the acceptance of encountering your own vulnerability as you experience the fragility of human life. And so it also requires courage to enter in the patient's experience of the dying process through being present. Courage helps you avoid filling up what may be perceived as empty spaces to give room for silence.

"Courage helps you avoid filling up what may be perceived as empty spaces to give room for silence."

Helping Family Members to Be Present

In a systematic review of literature on families in end-of-life care, Andershed (2006) addressed themes of how family members were open to the dying patient's world. Family members wanted to be with their dying relative, they wanted to be present when the relative died, and they wanted the opportunity to say "Goodbye." Family members also used time to learn what was important to their dying relative and to find a way to fulfill those wishes if possible. This led to feelings of relief for the relatives. They experienced peaceful times, but also hardship in managing the responsibilities of both daily life and preparing for the loss of a family member.

You can help family members understand what it means to be present for their dying relative. Listening may be as important as doing, silence *can* be meaningful, and spending time with their dying relative is important. It's also important, however, for them to make adequate time for their own rest and sustenance. Look for ways to make it easier for relatives to comfortably spend time with a dying relative in what may be a busy health care environment. Finally, although it is highly encouraged and desirable on the part of family members to be present when the moment of death occurs, it is not always possible. After all, few can predict when the actual moment will occur. If relatives miss the moment of death, you may need to help them work through their guilt, regret, or anger that may result from missing the moment of death.

Developing the Art of Nursing Presence

To be present with patients in the dying process, patients must invite you into their world, which does not happen without mutuality. This means that you must also invite patients and their family members into your world.

A nurse learns presence by being present (Doona et al., 1997). Being present involves the use of self. Osterman and Schwartz-Barcott (1996) conceptualized four levels of presence:

- Physical presence

- Partial presence

- Full presence

- Transcendent presence

Full presence and transcendent presence are most consistent with what it means to be truly present with a patient. Full presence means that you offer physical and psychological presence to meet patients' needs for comfort and support. Transcendent presence, the highest level, is more spiritual in nature. A patient may feel a connectedness with a nurse that contributes to positive emotion and a reduction in anxiety. Snyder and Lindquist (2000) describe "centering" as a strategy to help you learn to be present. To center on your patient, you pause before entering the patient's room and repeat the patient's name. This allows you to focus attention on the patient and reduce distractions outside the patient's experience. Two important precursors or antecedents to developing presence are:

1. A trusting relationship between you and a patient who needs facilitation of life processes.

2. A desire to help, connection with the patient, willingness to be vulnerable to the experience of the patient, and self-confidence (Snyder & Lindquist, 2000).

The intention to develop the key elements of nursing presence—attentiveness, accountability, sensitivity, openness, and active listening—will help you build "presencing" skills. Being present is not passive. It requires doing (Stanley, 2002). Presence does not necessarily mean finding more time; it is more about the willingness to focus on really being there during the time you have. Melnechenko (2003) speaks of the gift of "welcoming presence" that helps others to make sense of their experience and seek quality of life. The nurse who has learned the art of being present will facilitate quality of life for patients who are facing the end of their lives.

Reflective Practice

Being fully present involves deliberate attention to actions and behaviors that facilitate presence. Knowledge about the meaning of presence, how it occurs, and strategies for facilitating presence all contribute to development of presencing skills.

"We may struggle with the tension of what it means to be a professional and what are appropriate boundaries in our interactions with patients and families about the very sensitive and significant life event of death."

Our own characteristics and attitudes, however, may create challenges to being fully present. Nursing work does not seem consistent with the meaning of being present. Most nurses are focused on "doing" and "fixing problems." If we are successful, we feel rewarded for our accomplishment. We then move on to the next thing we need to do. In a sense, being present stops the flow of action. In being present, we may not feel like we are "doing" something. Being present also may not feel like we are "fixing" something. However, when we nurture the elements of nursing presence in our interactions—attentiveness, accountability, sensitivity, openness, and active listening—we are creating an environment that can help patients and families "fix" their experiences. Patients and families may come to a new understanding of the dying experience that involves acceptance, peace, closure, or meaningful communication. You may gain new insights about patient and family needs and interventions that could be helpful. These nursing insights are based on understanding the uniqueness of patients and families' experiences and are not based on your understanding of a set of nursing diagnoses and interventions commonly associated with dying patients. The ability to be present and create presence in working with dying patients and families is a high level of communication competence. Nursing action takes on a different meaning in intervening to be present.

We may also encounter tension as we strive to be fully present. Our meaning of self may be challenged as we work to encounter the patient as unique and having something to teach us. We need to take off our masks of being the experts. Yes, we do have a knowledge base and experience, but we need a patient's guidance in telling us how to use that knowledge base. Being present involves the use of self. As nurses, we are also unique, which means use of self will not be the same for every nurse, nor will it be the same with each patient. This means that what one nurse does to be fully present may not work for another nurse. We may struggle with the tension of what it means to be a professional and what boundaries are appropriate in our interactions with patients and families about the very sensitive and significant life event of death. Reflecting on these tensions that may lead to ethical conflict can help us work toward choosing the right way to be a good nurse.

Ethical Practice in Being Present

Ethical Problem: *How can I be present for dying patients and family members when there are many demands for my time and attention?*

What should I value?
- Autonomy of others.
- Uniqueness of each person—patients, family members, and health care staff.
- Importance of all aspects of care: physical, psychosocial, and spiritual.
- Knowledge and contributions of health care team members.

What should I be?
- Compassionate.
- Authentic.
- Competent.
- A professional who maintains appropriate boundaries and honors confidentiality.

What should I do?
- Relegate power associated with expert role to the sidelines.
- Center focus on patient.
- Let go of the need to "fix" the situation.
- Work with interdisciplinary health care team to plan strategies and time for development of "presencing" skills.

Nurses' Stories

Attentiveness

When we walk into a patient's room or into a patient's home, we need to center ourselves on the patient and family. Sometimes it's difficult to pay full attention to what is going on around us—particularly if we are busy, uncomfortable with the situation, or preoccupied.

An experienced home care-hospice nurse observed:

> I learned my lesson the day I walked into the home of a dying woman. Her daughter was caring for her and in obvious distress over her mother's condition. While I concentrated on the patient—taking her blood pressure, assessing her lungs, checking her bladder for distention—the daughter hovered. Neither of us noticed the daughter's 2-year-old in the background until he started choking on a button. We were able to get it dislodged, but after that, whenever I walked into a home, I paid attention to all the family members.

Another home care-hospice nurse explained how she gives her full attention to patients and family members:

> To symbolize the importance of being present with a patient and his or her family and to assume my given role, it was helpful for me to visualize the symbolic act of removing my "sandals" (shoes) at the threshold of my patient's door as well as removing my "crown" (hat, sweater/coat, and so on). This reminded me that I was a guest in my patient's home and to visualize my professional service to my patient.

Accountability

This means thinking about what is right for a patient and family from their point of view and being willing to learn from them.

A pediatric oncology nurse related the story of a young girl with leukemia:

> All the tests looked good and the doctors wanted to discharge her to home.
> No one, including me, was listening to the little girl who kept saying,
> "Something is wrong. I know something is wrong." Just as we were getting
> her ready to be discharged, she collapsed with peritonitis. She knew and we
> weren't listening.

Sensitivity, Openness, and Active Listening

In working with dying patients and their families, we must always be aware of
the patient and family's experience at that moment in time. We must be open to
entering into their world and listening carefully to what they say and what they
understand.

A palliative care nurse recounted her experience in a large metropolitan teaching hospital with a 40-year-old farmer and his wife. The patient had advanced
testicular cancer with multiple complications. She sat with the patient and his
wife through a care conference led by the patient's oncologist.

> The oncologist stood at the foot of the bed and talked down to the patient.
> He explained in highly technical terms all the treatment possibilities. They
> would add TPN to his regimen; if he had trouble breathing, they would
> intubate him; they would monitor his potassium level; and so on and so
> forth.

> The patient's wife listened attentively. After the doctor finished his speech,
> he asked, "Any questions?" No one said anything, so the doctor left the
> room. After he left, I sat quietly with them for a few moments. After a
> minute or two of silence, I asked, "Do you understand what's going on
> here?" The wife looked at at me with tears in her eyes and asked, "Does
> this mean he can go home? He really wants to go home." Ever since then, I
> have been very aware of how easy it is for us to put up a barrier in difficult
> situations by using technical terms and by lecturing rather than listening.

Key Points

- **Take time to center yourself.** Focus on a patient's unique situation. A hospice-home care nurse advises, "Before I walk up to the door, I spend a few moments in the car reflecting on the patient and family. Then I close my eyes and take a deep breath and let my mind go blank."

- **Be aware of your physical presence and your physical surroundings.** A palliative care nurse working in a hospital notes, "Too often I see nurses 'hugging the charts' and standing at the foot of the bed when they talk with patients. This behavior sends the message to the patient that 'I'm not open to what you have to say.' Whenever possible, I sit near the head of the bed and leave my paperwork on my lap."

- **Be comfortable with silence.** A hospice nurse says, "I've learned to carry tissues with me and to sit quietly if my patients need to cry. Sometimes I cry with them."

- **Listen to what patients and families are saying.** A hospital nurse advises, "Sometimes it's hard to really listen. Especially when you are busy and your mind is full of tasks. When this happens to me, I take a moment to re-center myself. Sometimes, I will sit down. Sitting beside a patient can be more important than making sure the sheets are properly tucked in."

- **Take time to care for yourself.** Be aware that you can't be all things to all people. Reflect with your team members on the rewards and challenges of caregiving experiences. A hospice nurse said, "I couldn't do this job if it wasn't for the other people on my team."

REFLECTION QUESTIONS

1. In the previous scenario of the care conference among the doctor, the farmer, his wife, and the nurse, what would you do to be fully present with the patient and wife? How could you use attentiveness, accountability, sensitivity, openness, and active listening to be fully present?

2. What skills and abilities do you need to develop to become competent in being present? What will you do to develop these skills and abilities?

3. From an ethical perspective, how should you, as the nurse, respond to the physician's behavior? Consider the well-being of the patient, physician, and health care organization.

References

Andershed, B. (2006). Relatives in end-of-life care. Part 1: A systematic review of the literature in the five last years, January 1999-February 2004. *Journal of Clinical Nursing, 15*(9), 1158-1169.

Benner, P. (1984). *From novice to expert: Excellence and power in clinical nursing practice.* Menlo Park, CA: Addison-Wesley.

Borne, K. (2001). Communication with dying patients and family members: A body, mind, and spirit approach. In B. Poor & Gail P. Poirrier, (Eds.), *End of life nursing care* (pp. 227-236). Sudbury, MA: Jones and Bartlett.

Boston, P., Towers, A., & Barnard, D. (2001). Embracing vulnerability: Risk and empathy in palliative care. *Journal of Palliative Care, 17*(4), 248-253.

Brown, L. (1986). The experience of care: Patient perspectives. *Topics in Clinical Nursing, 8,* 56-62.

Doona, M. E., Haggerty, L. A., & Chase, S. K. (1997). Nursing presence: An existential exploration of the concept. *Scholarly Inquiry for Nursing Practice, 11,* 3-16.

Edwards, P. (2005). An overview of end-of-life discussion. *International Journal of Palliative Nursing, 11*(1), 21-27.

Gardner, D. (1985). Presence. In G. Bulecheck & J. McClosky (Eds.), *Nursing interventions: Treatments for nursing diagnosis* (pp. 316-324). Philadelphia: Saunders.

Melnechenko, K. L. (2003). To make a difference: Nursing presence. *Nursing Forum, 38*(2), 18-24.

Minick, P. (1995). The power of human caring: Early recognition of patient problems. *Scholarly Inquiry for Nursing Practice, 9*, 303-317.

Osterman, P., & Schwartz-Barcott, D. (1996). Presence: Four ways of being there. *Nursing Forum, 31*(2), 23-30.

Parse, R. R. (1992). Human becoming: Parse's theory of nursing. *Nursing Science Quarterly, 5*, 35-42.

Pettigrew, J. (1990). International nursing care: The ministry of presence. *Critical Care Nursing Clinics of North America, 2*, 503-508.

Snyder, M., Brandt, C.L., & Tseng, Y. (2000). Measuring intervention outcomes: Impact of nurse characteristics. *International Journal of Human Caring, 5*(3), 36-42.

Snyder, M., & Lindquist, R. (2000).Use of presence in the critical care unit. *AACN Clinical Issues, 11*, 27-33.

Stanley, K. J. (2000). Silence is not golden: Conversations with the dying. *Clinical Journal of Oncology Nursing, 4*(1), 34-40.

Stanley, K. J. (2002). The healing power of presence: Respite from the fear of abandonment. *Oncology Nursing Forum, 29*(6), 935-940.

Travelbee, J. (1966. *Interpersonal aspects of nursing.* Philadelphia: F. A. Davis.

Zerwehk, J. V. (2006). *Nursing care at the end of life.* Philadelphia: F. A. Davis.

In hospice, sometimes I feel like we think we have all the answers. If only we spoke openly and honestly to patients, then everybody would embrace the fact that they're dying. I've come to realize, though, that people don't want to be dead. They want pain relief and all of that, but they really would prefer not to be dead. I work with this wonderful chaplain who taught me to be attached to the journey, not the outcome. It has been my saving grace in staying sane in some of these situations where you look at what's going on, and the demands being made by the families and patients about the kind of care they're getting, and you're saying, "Oh, my ... why would you even want to go through this personally or have a loved one go through this?" And then you realize it's not my journey, it's their journey. It's their experience; it's what they need to have happen. It's being with patients and families, giving them information, clarifying, speaking honestly and sensitively, but understanding that they are going to do what they need to do. Again, it's not the outcome, it's the process.

—Hospice nurse

2

•

Knowing What to Say and When to Say It

To know what to say and when to say it, we must recognize that communicating with patients and families at the end of life is both an art and a process. The first step in developing the art is to recognize that dying is a unique journey for each patient and each family.

Best Communication Practices in End-of-Life Care

The National Consensus Project for Quality Palliative Care (2004) identifies communication skills as one of the core elements of palliative care. Communication skills that are particularly relevant to caring for patients who are dying include the following:

- Effectively sharing information in a developmentally appropriate manner—being sensitive to cognitive and emotional abilities.

- Actively listening to patients and families.

- Assisting patients and families in determining goals.

- Effectively communicating with health care team members.

In addition to effective communication, the American Association of Colleges of Nursing (2008) competency for facilitating a peaceful death includes the concept of compassionate communication, which emphasizes both empathy and concern for suffering.

Why Communication Is Important at the End of Life

Hearing, interpreting meaning, and applying information to your life situation are especially challenging when faced with the knowledge that you are dying. At the same time, health professionals have their own language—lingo and jargon—and may retreat to the safety of that language in an attempt to communicate difficult information to patients.

In one report, 50% of families with a relative hospitalized in an intensive care unit (ICU) did not understand physicians' communications about diagnosis, prognosis, or treatment options (Azoulay et al., 2000). Patients are more likely to share physical concerns than psychosocial concerns. Nondisclosure of concerns, including those in the psychosocial realm, is related to increased distress for dying patients (Heaven & Maguire, 1998).

For dying people, the world becomes smaller—often they can focus only on their illness and a few important relationships. If they don't talk about their experience, they are more likely to feel lonely, isolated, and abandoned. They may interpret a lack of discussion about their situation as a lack of care (Callahan & Kelly, 1992).

When communication is effective, patients are more likely to identify their most important feelings and needs about their situations. This helps them cope with bad news, make treatment decisions, and keep better track of both desired and adverse responses to treatment and care (Maguire, 1999). With a repertoire of effective communication skills, nurses will be able to address the common concerns of patients who are dying, such as loss of control and anxiety about what will happen, fear of dying, what to do about their pain and other discomforts, and how to make a decision about their treatment (Pollard & Swift, 1999).

Characteristics of Effective Communication

Nurses who are compassionate, comprehensive, clear, honest, and timely in their communication with patients, family members, and health care staff will contribute to good end-of-life care (Ciccarello, 2003; Kirk, Kirk, & Kristjanson, 2004; Miettinen, Alaviuhkola, & Pietial, 2001; Pierce, 1999). The environment for communication should be one that is private, provides enough time to reflect on and discuss information and feelings, minimizes interruptions, and includes the presence of important support persons (Dahlin & Giansiracusa, 2006; Moore, 2005). Getting to know one another and providing opportunities for normal, everyday discussions help to build trust among nurses, patients, and families.

"Patients are encouraged to tell their stories of life and illness, helping them to transform the chaos in their lives to acceptance."

Storytelling can be effective for communicating meaning and the emotions connected with encountering death (Pollard & Swift, 1999). A Brazilian palliative-care ambulatory clinic uses a storytelling approach both as a teaching tool and therapeutic intervention. Patients are encouraged to tell their stories of life and illness, helping them to transform the chaos in their lives to acceptance. Videotaping, audiotaping, or journaling might provide a way for patients to tell their stories. As health professionals listen to the stories of their patients, their expressions of empathy and compassion assist patients in creating a new script that helps them to overcome and transcend death (DeBendetto, deCastro, deCarvalho, Sanogo, & Blasco, 2007).

Choosing a time for communication often depends on patient and family receptivity and nurse availability. However, some situations in end-of-life nursing care require a more urgent response to communicating with patients and family members. You should facilitate more immediate communication when death is imminent, the patient is talking about wanting to die, the family asks about hospice, the patient is suffering and has a poor prognosis, or hospitalization is needed for severe and progressive illness (Dahlin & Giansiracusa, 2006).

Barriers to Communication

Communication barriers in end-of-life care may be related to blocks the nurse creates, patient characteristics, or societal factors. In one study, nurses in a focus group suggested that a lack of time, lack of experience, emotional exhaustion, and assumptions about patients not wanting to talk about death all contributed to the inability to be effective communicators (Clarke & Ross, 2006). Specific behaviors of nurses that prevent open and direct discussion between nurse and patient include

- physically distancing yourself from the patient;

- ignoring emotional cues such as tears or statements of sadness;

- focusing on physical tasks, changing the subject, and giving false reassurance that everything will be okay; and

- gatekeeping or withholding information (Andershed, 2006; Pollard & Swift, 1999).

A lack of knowledge about common concerns and problems patients experience at the end of life and poor assessment skills will also inhibit the communication process between nurses and patients (Pollard & Swift, 1999). "Ignorers," those who fail to recognize patient cues about problems and concerns, and "informers," those who are busy giving explanations or advice, will block important communication needed for planning nursing care (Perrin, 2006).

Health professionals may hold certain values that interfere with their own openness and freedom to address dying more directly. They may value being stoic or strong, fear emotional vulnerability, fear death, or may simply be unaware of their beliefs and values because they avoid confronting and reflecting on their own experiences and responses to death (Pollard & Swift, 1999).

Patients may also inhibit communication if they are hesitant to share their concerns, have communication style preferences that are not matched by the nurse, have cultural differences in communication patterns (see Chapter 8), or are not able or ready to confront death. In their attempt to cope with the prospect of being near death, patients and families may use defense mechanisms such as anger and denial that repel any communication attempts from nurses (Clarke & Ross, 2006; Perrin, 2006; Pollard & Swift, 1999).

Finally, death has become more hidden in hospitals and institutions. In Western societies, we tend to use language about death that is less direct, such as "passed away" or "gone to a better place" (Clarke & Hanson, 2001). In Norway, a great majority of health professionals and family members were reluctant to discuss an expected death with the patient, although the healthy elders who were interviewed said they would like to discuss their wishes before "the time has come." Death is a difficult topic in our current society, and it may seem that it is easier to avoid the topic until death is imminent. However, the goal of a peaceful death is more likely to be reached if patient, family, and health care team can effectively discuss expectations, needs, and wishes in a comfortable environment with adequate time, attention, and sensitivity.

Sharing Information

Sharing information with patients and families is an art that involves understanding several criteria. The discussion should be

- desired by the patient;
- timely;
- accurate;
- understandable;
- gentle, respectful, and compassionate (Latimer, 1998).

For example, before sharing specific information, we should determine what the patient already knows about their situation and what kind of information is desired. If the information is bad news, use very simple language and allow time for silence so that the patient can absorb the information and ask questions (Perrin, 2006). Information needs to be in real-time and not delayed, unless patient cues clearly indicate the timing is wrong (Miettinen et al., 2001). Tell the patient you know it is difficult to hear the information and ask if it is okay to discuss. Talk about symptom management; clarify the patient's understanding about resuscitation and advance directives; and provide information about resources such as chaplain, palliative consult, and hospice services (Forest, 2004).

Provide written information when it is available. Always clarify the patient's understanding and provide a time for questions. Come back later, if possible, for a face-to-face or phone visit to respond to concerns and answer additional questions.

Remember that other factors affect patients' abilities to absorb important information. Anxiety resulting from disturbing or traumatic communications will reduce the amount of information that is heard and processed. Also, educational development level, stress levels, physical limitations, sleep deprivation, and language barriers influence understanding and the ability to apply information (Perrin, 2006).

In a systematic review of the literature on family members' needs for information, Andershed (2006) found that family members feared not getting enough information and described "being in the dark" when they lacked information. Family members had greater satisfaction with care when they understood the care and why it was being given (Rogers, Karlsen, & Addington-Hall, 2000). This knowledge also helped family members to be more effective caregivers. Topics of information can include

- the patient's diagnosis and condition, and what to expect in illness progression;

- what is being done for the patient;

- current and expected symptoms and effective treatment for relief of symptoms;

- helpful resources and how to obtain them;

- how to make decisions, and how to plan and prepare for care (Andershed, 2006; Dahlin & Giansiracusa, 2006).

"Three critical factors for building trust were flexibility, continuity, and empowerment of family members."

At the same time, nurses will need to recognize that patients and their family members may have differing needs for amount of information (Andrade, 2006). This means that sensitivity to timing is important. An assessment of a person's readiness for information will help to determine timely sharing of information without giving information that patients or family members will consider to be too late.

What to Say: Questions to Ask

Patient

Would it be okay to talk about this now?

What have you been told?

What are your greatest concerns?

What is it like for you right now?

How are you doing with this?

What really matters for you right now?

What information do you need right now?

How are you getting your support?

Whom would you like to be involved in your care and decision-making?

Is there anything else you were hoping we would talk about today?

What are your hopes?

What gives you meaning in life?

If you were to die soon, what would be left undone?

Is there some event that would add a great deal of meaning to your life?

Are there things you need to do in case things don't go as well as we hope?

Family

What has the patient told you about his or her situation or wishes?

What similar situations has your family been through?

Andrade, 2006; Dahlin & Giansiracusa, 2006, p. 76; Forest, 2004, p. 273; Perrin, 2006, p. 30; Weaver, 2004, p. 523; Zerwekh, 2006, p. 119.

Creating Relationships

The existence of a trusting relationship enhances effectiveness of communication between nurses and patients and between nurses and family members. Analysis of a case study about building trust between a palliative care team and the family of a dying patient revealed that the three critical factors for building trust were flexibility, continuity, and empowerment of family members (Holmberg, 2006). Nurses were deliberate about giving messages that supported family-member choices to live their everyday lives as normally as possible. This required flexibility from the palliative care team. Presence and time were both viewed as contributing to a sense of continuity in caregiving. The palliative care team created a "patient-centered, rapid-cycle" feedback loop that improved the quality of care. This strategy resulted in timely, frequent communication that validated the messages. In addition, the case study analysis showed that time for "small talk" actually provided opportunities for evaluating care and involving family caregivers in identifying needed changes.

Green's (2006) description of a therapeutic relationship includes many of the elements that define being present with patients:

- active listening

- silence and nonverbal communication

- therapeutic touch

Some verbal responses facilitate development of a therapeutic relationship. These include:

- paraphrasing,

- asking open-ended questions to encourage sharing of concerns and feelings,

- summarizing to patients what you hear them say (Green, 2006).

In the person-centered counseling approach described by Green, you use the relationship to encourage positive change and growth in someone who has experienced a traumatic event. The goals of a person-centered counseling approach are to help meet patients' needs of self-actualization (a sense of competence to deal with their problems and emotions) and to be loved and valued by others. This approach to relationship development assumes that a patient wants to develop a relationship and that everyone has the potential for growth and change.

A therapeutic relationship requires an accepting, empathetic, nonjudgmental, warm, and genuine response from the nurse (Green, 2006); however, the nurse also needs to maintain professional boundaries. In some situations, patients may have expectations of friendship, and it is up to the nurse to be alert to possible red flags concerning boundaries. To be genuine, it is important to know yourself and respond with authenticity, and have no pretense based on role or expertise. It is difficult to remove all inequity, because hierarchy already exists in a relationship between one person who is ill and vulnerable and the other who is healthy and has expert knowledge for responding to the needs of the vulnerable person (Green). This inequity can be diminished by acknowledging and respecting the expert knowledge of patients regarding their own wants and needs and inviting them to share that knowledge in decision-making.

What to Say: Words and Strategies

Words

I am sorry. I have some bad news for you.

Because we cannot cure your illness, I want you to know we will continue to care for you and support you.

Accepting such a serious illness must be difficult, because you have taken such good care of yourself.

I know that making a decision about this is extremely painful, but if you don't make plans now, you may lose that chance.

Strategies

Allow distressed patients to tell the story of their trauma and to cry to release emotion.

Be cautious about offering advice. It is best to help patients talk through concerns, so they can think about the different options.

Use paraphrases (not word-for-word quotes) to validate your understanding of the essence of the communication.

Acknowledge intense emotions to show care and validation for the relevance of feelings.

Summarize important themes to reassure patients and family members that their concerns are understood.

Use humor or lighthearted talk for a short period if you believe it might help create an atmosphere that is more comfortable for disclosing concerns.

Avoid health care jargon, as this distances patients and families.

Avoid multitasking.

Do not delay discussion because of your own discomfort. Once patients become un-responsive, they lose the ability to determine the kind of end-of-life care they want.

Block, 2001, p. 953; Forest, 2004, p. 273; Moore, 2005; Perrin, 2006, p. 223; Radziewicz & Baile, 2001, p. 952; Wright, 2003.

Communication Needs Across the Lifespan

Individual development level is an important variable in the capacity for under-standing death. Nurses can use knowledge about levels of understanding and common concerns related to age group to tailor communication strategies to the developmental needs of patients. Although some generalizations can be made about communication needs based on age group, assessing a person's capacity for understanding and readiness for communication is necessary. Skill in communi-cating with families is essential when caring for dying children or adolescents. See Table 2.1 for common concerns and suggestions for communication with people in specific age groups.

Table 2.1   Communication Based on Age Group

Working with children

- Share information based on the child's ability to absorb that information.
- Consider that children are often insulated from death; their experience may be based on television or movies, rather than real life.
- Children younger than 7 may not understand the permanence of death.

- Children older than 7 often understand the permanence of death and that they could die from their illness.
- Explain how illness will affect the child's life.
- Children may be able to work through emotions in play, art, and music therapy.
- Consider that sharing your own emotions may burden the family.

Working with adolescents

- Adolescents generally respond well to truthful and direct communication.
- Consider making a contract specifying that you agree to share important information and the adolescent will ask questions.
- Adolescents generally have the capacity to verbalize the meaning of illness and death to themselves and the effect on others.
- Spend some time with the adolescent alone without the parent present, because the adolescent may be reluctant to verbalize fears in the presence of a parent.
- Adolescents over 14 are assumed to have capacity to make medical decisions.

Working with young and middle-age adults

- Encourage identification of any unfinished business and unresolved relationships, and discuss possible strategies for responding to these needs.
- Facilitate expression of emotions such as anger, fear, and disappointment.
- Help a dying parent to identify strategies for saying goodbye to young children, such as leaving words or mementos for their future.

Working with older adults

- Avoid assuming the older person has led a full life and is ready to die.
- Provide time for life review (see Chapter 3).
- Encourage discussion of fears and what can be done to alleviate fears.
- Assist in identifying short-term goals that enhance quality of life.
- Avoid "shielding" older adults from a terminal diagnosis.
- Invite participation in treatment decisions.

Sources: Ashurst, 2007; Clarke & Ross, 2006; Freyer, 2004; Newson, 2003; Perrin, 2006.

Interdisciplinary Strategies

Having health care team members "on the same page" in working toward common goals in palliative care is important. Mixed messages resulting from different philosophies of care can confuse patients and prevent them from working through their concerns and making decisions based on consistent information (Clarke & Ross, 2006).

"Nurses often think of death as a natural process, while physicians often perceive it as failure."

Physicians and nurses may hold different values that influence their communication with patients. Nurses often think of death as a natural process, while physicians often perceive it as failure (Clarke & Ross, 2006). A "rescue culture" might exist in ICUs, making creation of an environment that supports a "good death" difficult. Finding time for busy physicians and nurses to discuss strategies for helping patients and families through the dying process is challenging. However, effective multidisciplinary communication is essential for high-quality end-of-life care.

Formal communication structures can create an environment for successful interdisciplinary communication (Boyle, Miller, & Forbes-Thompson, 2005). One strategy is to schedule a multidisciplinary meeting within 72 hours of admission for any patient at risk of dying. The first meeting should focus on medical condition and treatment options, the patient's understanding and wishes, the plan of care, and a way to determine the success of the plan of care. Later meetings can focus on meeting palliative care needs. This type of intervention has resulted in fewer days in the ICU and an earlier start to palliative care (Boyle et al.).

Another model is to create a physician and clinical nurse specialist (CNS) team to focus on families of patients who have a high risk of dying. The physician provides daily medical updates and offers treatment guidelines. The CNS gives daily information, clarifies communication and understanding, listens to family concerns, and explains what the family wants to know. This strategy has led to shorter ICU and hospital stays and lower cost of care.

Instituting daily team-consensus procedures is a third model for strengthening interdisciplinary communication. Team members meet daily to come to consensus about goals of care, resulting in improved communication and decision-making.

Strategies for Improving Communication

A survey of nurses revealed that most were confident about the physical care they provided, but they did not have the same level of confidence about discussing death with patients (McDonnell, Johnson, Gallagher, & McGlade, 2002). We need to be intentional about developing communication skills for talking with patients and families about death and dying. We can cultivate our own attitudes that support skill development in effective communication strategies, such as being less anxious about death and responding with unconditional positive regard for patients and families (Wilkinson, 1998).

Strategies for improving communication in end-of-life care include the following:

- Take small steps.
- Make a specific improvement plan.
- Develop organizational strategies.

An example of a small step is observing a more experienced nurse (Forest, 2004). This can increase your knowledge of possible words and phrases to use that arise naturally while giving care. You can choose from many options to include in a communication-improvement plan. These include arranging for structured supervision, keeping a diary, asking for peer support, discussing specific cases, and attending structured educational sessions (Pollard & Swift, 1999).

Wilkinson (1998) evaluated an intensive education program to improve communication during end-of-life care. The program was six months in length, involved 26 hours of skills and attitude training, and included individual feedback sessions.

Communication areas that were most challenging for the nurses were emotionally laden topics such as

- patients' awareness of diagnosis or prognosis,

- responding to difficult questions,

- conducting a psychological assessment,

- dealing with patient and family emotions.

Self-awareness and self-reflection are essential for any communication improvement program. In addition to education targeted to improve communication strategies, organizations can develop or find specific screening tools that will assist nurses with psychosocial assessment of patients and families and arrange for mentorship in communication skill-building.

Reflective Practice

Although our nursing education helps us learn how to use therapeutic communication, a taboo exists for many of us when it comes to talking about death. Our culture celebrates youth and energy. We may experience a sense of uneasiness or anxiety as we attempt to make the connection with patients and families to talk about death and dying. Saying the "right thing" is what we strive to do. We also want to say the right thing in a way that is comfortable for our own context of understanding death and dying. How do we do this while also maintaining our professional boundaries? How do we avoid giving advice? Death moves us into our own emotional realm, because it is such a significant life event. Being with patients and families at such a vulnerable, significant time calls for a response that is professional, but it also may generate close emotional connections.

We should not hold back from those close emotional connections that can help patients and families to prepare for death and find comfort during the dying process. However, reflecting on our actions and patients and families' responses is important to determine that we are meeting *their* emotional needs and not just our own. Certainly, working with patients and families who are encountering end-of-life issues and decisions can be very rewarding for nurses. This kind of satisfaction is motivating and prevents burnout. However, if we are focused on meeting our own needs, we will miss important opportunities for communicating with patients and families.

"We can journey with them, but our patients must also find their own way."

The temptation exists to tell patients and families what they need to do to prepare for dying. We can journey with them, but our patients must also find their own way. We can educate, offer options, discuss approaches, contact resources, and work with our colleagues to present a unified approach, but we cannot determine the right way to approach death for our patients and their families. The virtues of patience and courage are important for knowing what to say and when to say it. Courage in end-of-life dialogue sometimes may mean taking a risk to see what a person's response might be. Our efforts may be met with anger or distancing. We must keep in mind that talking about death and dying with others is a learning process. We can always pull back from questions or dialogue and say, "I am available when you find it is important to talk."

We also must be open to understanding the different values and perspectives held by our nursing and interdisciplinary colleagues as we work together to care for dying patients and their families. We know that "getting on the same page" is necessary for continuity in approach and is a best practice for communicating with dying patients and their family members. Respecting our colleagues, asking questions to encourage dialogue, and sharing our own opinions about approaches to use in talking with patients and families can help us work toward achieving effective communication with our colleagues. We can also embody the virtues of courage and patience as we interact with our colleagues to develop a consensus about best practices in working with patients and families at the end of life.

Ethical Practice in What to Say and When

ETHICAL PROBLEM: *What should I do when decisions need to be made for a patient and family to prepare for death, but they do not want to talk about it?*

What should I value?

- Understanding patient and family member perspectives.
- Using best practices in end-of-life communication and caregiving.
- Assisting patients and family members in making decisions to meet their desires for end-of- life care.

Who should I be?

- A courageous nurse who is willing to talk about difficult subjects.
- An accountable nurse who provides ongoing opportunities for patient and family communication about end-of-life choices.
- A nurse who is patient and sensitive to timing and to the process that patients and family members are experiencing.

What should I do?

- Talk with interdisciplinary team members through a formal communication structure to develop a consensus on approach to communication and recommended care strategies.
- Explain to patients and family members that you are available to talk about their concerns and worries.
- Explain to patients and family members that it is important to talk about decisions that need to be made soon and offer a choice about who should be present and when the discussion should take place.
- Ask open-ended questions to encourage initial discussions.

Nurses' Stories

Communicating When Time Is of the Essence

Knowing what to say and when to say it involves assessing a person's situation, understanding the information needs of that person, and communicating in a way that is understandable. We don't always have the luxury of time to build a relationship with patients and their families, but we can still communicate with them in ways that convey compassion and attention to their needs.

An ICU nurse talks about having very little time with the husband of a dying patient who was on a ventilator.

> As an ICU nurse, I often walk into situations where I don't know the patient or the family, and they are in an acute crisis of some sort. In this case, I hadn't seen the physicians yet, but I knew they had been working with the patient for quite some time, and the decision had been made to take the patient off the ventilator. The husband came in and I asked him, "Is this what your wife wants?" He said, "Yes." I replied, "I'm sorry that I haven't met you. I realize what your wife has said and what she wants, but I also know through my experience that if we do this today, she's not going to live very long." And he said, "Oh, no one's told me that." I asked, "Is there anybody else you want here?" And he said, "Oh, yes. I need some time to call them in." If I hadn't been straightforward with him, he would not have had the time to bring his family together to say goodbye to his wife.

Communicating When a Patient Is Angry

The art of communicating with patients sometimes involves getting beyond their anger or other reactions to the situation. A CNS on a medical surgical unit talks about an extremely angry patient:

> He was very sick, and the physician wanted to keep him in the hospital over the weekend to make sure he was stable before going home. The patient was so angry about it that no one wanted to go into his room—including me. I finally took a deep breath and sat down to talk with him. I asked him a few questions, but mainly I listened. His anger finally subsided, and he said, "I know I'm very sick, but I promised my daughter I would be at her wedding this weekend. I don't want to break my promise." Until then, no one had explored why he was so insistent on going home. We arranged for a day pass, and he was able to attend the wedding.

Communicating When the Patient and Family Don't Want to Talk

As nurses, we are often challenged by situations in which family members assume their relative does not know that death is likely. In these situations, the dying person, who often knows he or she is dying, may assume that family members do not want to talk. No one knows how to begin the conversation. We know that the dying person and family members will likely benefit from opening their communication, but we struggle with how to facilitate that communication. A Norwegian home care nurse explained how she worked with a family to begin the conversation.

> I've also [had] situations where I've spoken to relatives who won't discuss it, because they don't want to depress the patient. So, you talk to the patient alone, and the patient says that his wife won't discuss it. When you talk to her alone, she says that he doesn't know that he's dying. Then, I've actually gone in and convinced everyone to sit down and discuss it. I've started a conversation with the patient with the point of view of asking him to be honest with himself. I ask if he feels, perhaps, that the situation's a little more difficult than the impression he gives. If I feel I can say that, which in this particular situation I did ... everybody started talking. It was very difficult for the wife to hear it, because she was in shock that her husband realized how ill he was. But in a way, it made things much easier, because then she could start talking to him about where they were in the situation. And he died much more relaxed.

Key Points

Communication with patients at the end of life often means conveying bad news or distressing information. Our own attitudes toward death and dying can contribute to a reluctance to talk with patients and families. We can create barriers by physically distancing ourselves, ignoring cues from our patients, or providing false reassurances. To be present in communication with our patients, we must

- Provide information that is timely, honest, and understandable.

- Communicate with compassion and empathy.

- Be patient, allow silence, and let the patient decide when to ask for more information.

- Encourage patients and families to tell their stories.

- Use the resources of the interdisciplinary team.

REFLECTION QUESTIONS

1. What fears, anxieties, concerns, or experiences with death could potentially create barriers in your communication with dying patients and their family members? What strategies can you use to overcome potential barriers?

2. How can you use the virtue of courage to help you initiate effective discussion with patients about their dying experiences?

3. What can you do and say to create a relationship that will facilitate communication with patients and family members at the end of life, when time is limited?

References

American Association of Colleges of Nursing. (2008). Peaceful death: Recommended competencies and curricular guidelines for end-of-life nursing care. Retrieved February 14, 2008, from http://www.aacn.nche.edu/Publications/deathfin.html.

Andershed, B. (2006). Relatives in end-of-life care – part 1: A systematic review of the literature in the five last years, January 1999-February 2004. *Journal of Clinical Nursing, 15*(9), 1158-1169.

Andrade, P. D. (2006). Effective communication in palliative care: A nurse's responsibility and privilege. *DNA Reporter, 31*(3), 16-18.

Ashurst, A. (2007). Palliative care: Effective communication. *Nursing & Residential Care, 9*(2), 66-68.

Azoulay, E., Cheveret, S., Leleu, G., Pochard, F., Barboteu, M., Adrie, C., et al. (2000). Half the families of intensive care unit patients experience inadequate communication with physicians. *Critical Care Medicine, 28*, 3044-3049.

Block, S. (2001). Pyschological considerations, growth, and transcendence at the end of life: The art of the possible. *JAMA, 285*, 2898-2904.

Boyle, D. K., Miller, P. A., & Forbes-Thompson, S. A. (2005). Communication and end-of-life care in the intensive care unit: Patient, family, and clinician outcomes. *Critical Care Nursing Quarterly*, *28*(4), 302-316.

Callahan, M., & Kelley, P. (1992). *Final gifts: Understanding the special awareness, needs, and communications of the dying*. New York: Bantam.

Ciccarello, G. P. (2003). Strategies to improve end-of-life care in the intensive care unit. *Dimensions of Critical Care Nursing*, *22*(5), 216-222.

Clarke, A., & Hanson, E. (2001). Death and dying: Changing the culture of care. In A. Warren, L., Warren, & M. Nolan (Eds.), *Care services for later life: Transformations and critiques* (pp. 204-218). London: Jessica Kingsley.

Clarke, A., & Ross, H. (2006). Influences on nurses' communications with older people at the end of life: Perceptions and experiences of nurses working with palliative care and general medicine. *International Journal of Older People*, *1*, 34-43.

Dahlin, C. M., & Giansiracusa, D. F. (2006). Communication in palliative care. In B. R. Ferrell & N. Coyle (Eds.), *Textbook of palliative care nursing* (pp. 67-93). New York: Oxford University Press.

DeBendetto, M A. C., deCastro, A. G., deCarvalho, E., Sanogo, R., & Blasco, P. G. (2007). From suffering to transcendence. *Canadian Family Physician*, *53*, 1277-1279.

Forest, P. K. (2004). Being there: The essence of end-of-life nursing care. *Urologic Nursing*, *23*(4), 270-280.

Freyer, D. (2004). Care of the dying adolescent: Special considerations. *Pediatrics*, *113*, 381-388.

Green, A. (2006). A person-centered approach to palliative care nursing. *Journal of Hospice and Palliative Nursing*, *8*(5), 294-301.

Heaven, C., & Maguire, P. (1998). The relationship between patients' concerns and psychological distress in a hospice setting. *Psycho-Oncology*, *7*, 503-507.

Holmberg, L. (2006). Communication in action between family caregivers and a palliative care team. *Journal of Hospice and Palliative Nursing*, *8*(5), 276-287.

Kirk, P. Kirk, I., & Kristjanson, L. (2004). What do patients receiving palliative care for cancer and their families want to be told? A Canadian and Australian qualitative study. *British Medical Journal*, *328*, 1343-1349.

Latimer, E. (1998). Ethical care at the end of life. *Canadian Medical Association Journal*, *158*, 1741-1745.

Maguire, P. (1999). Improving communication with cancer patients. *European Journal of Cancer*, *35*(14), 2058-2065.

McDonnell, M., Johnson, D., Gallagher, A., & McGlade, K. (2002). Palliative care in district general hospitals: The nurse's perspective. *International Journal of Palliative Nursing, 8,* 160-175.

Miettinen, T., Alaviuhkola, H., & Pietial, A. (2001). The contribution of "good" palliative care to quality of life in dying patients: Family members' perceptions. *Journal of Family Nursing, 7*(3), 261-280.

Moore, C. D. (2005). Communication issues and advance care planning. *Seminars in Oncology Nursing, 21*(1), 11-19.

National Consensus Project for Quality Palliative Care (2004). *Clinical practice guidelines for quality palliative care.* Retrieved February 14, 2008, from http://www.nationalconsensusproject.org

Newson, P. (2003). How to support people during the process of dying. *Nursing & Residential Care, 5*(12), 556-563.

Perrin, K. O. (2006). Communicating with seriously ill and dying patients, their families, and their health care providers. In M. L. Matzo & D. W. Sherman (Eds.), *Palliative care nursing* (pp. 221-245). New York: Springer Publishing.

Pierce, S. F. (1999). Improving end-of-life care: Gathering questions from family members. *Nursing Forum, 34,* 5-14.

Pollard, A., & Swift, K. (1999). Communication skills in palliative care. In M. O'Connor & S. Aranda (Eds.), *Palliative care nursing: A guide to practice* (pp. 23-28). Melbourne, Australia: Ausmed.

Radziewicz, R., & Baile, W. F. (2001). Communication skills: Breaking bad news in the clinical setting. *Oncology Nursing Forum, 28,* 951-953.

Rogers, A., Karlsen, S., & Addington-Hall, J. (2000). All the services were excellent. It is when the human element comes in that things go wrong: Dissatisfaction with hospital care at the end of life. *Journal of Advanced Nursing, 31,* 768-774.

Weaver, A. W. (2004). Family health promotion during life-threatening illness at the end of life. In P. T. Bomar (Ed.), *Promoting health in families: Applying family research and theory to nursing practice* (pp. 507-533). Philadelphia: Saunders.

Wilkinson, S., Roberts, A., & Aldrige, J. (1998). Nurse-patient communication in palliative care: An evaluation of a communication skills programme. *Palliative Medicine, 12,* 13-22.

Wright, M. (2003). How to advise and support clients in the care home. *Nursing & Residential Care, 5*(7), 312-317.

Zerwekh, J. V. (2006). Nursing care at the end of life. Philadelphia: F.A. Davis.

*For my patients who are going through the trauma
and the chaos of dying, I consider hope to be a place
of rest for them. I don't see anything wrong with
them talking about going to the white sand beaches
in the Caribbean, even though I know they will
probably never get there. To dream and to wish and
to hope is human. My job is to be present with them
and to allow them their rest.*

—Hospice nurse

3

•

Responding to Patient and Family Wishes and Hopes

One of the biggest challenges to nurses in caring for dying patients and their families is to understand and honor wishes and hopes. This means recognizing their need for control and self-determination and eliciting their understanding of the meaning of a "good death." As a seasoned hospice nurse noted, "Sometimes I have to step back, take a deep breath, and put myself in my patient's shoes. Then I can start from where they are at."

In this chapter, we focus on communication strategies that consider the desires of patients and their family members as they struggle to work their way through the decision-making and coping with loss that are part of death.

Autonomy

Sometimes referred to as self-determination, autonomy means respecting the wishes of the patient and family. Supporting or promoting autonomy empowers patients and family members to make informed decisions about end-of-life care decisions (Coyle, 2006). Although following the principle of autonomy would mean that the patient's wishes are to be considered before the family's wishes, decisions about care at the end of life will affect and be affected by a patient's relationships (Ladd, Pasquella, & Smith, 2000). Autonomy is a strong European-American cultural value; other cultures may be more comfortable with a family-centered model of decision-making (Tilden, 1999). Interventions that are meant to support patient autonomy may not be well-received by patients and families who are not part of mainstream American culture. In interviews of hospitalized elders about their attitudes on having control over their end-of-life decisions, 27 preferred to have autonomy in their decisions, while 11 reported they would rather delegate the decision-making to their physicians, God, or fate (Kelner, 1995). Not everyone values autonomy equally. However, as an aging baby boomer population reaches the time of making end-of-life decisions, control over those decisions may be important for an increasing number of our patients.

"Sometimes I have to step back, take a deep breath, and put myself in my patient's shoes. Then I can start from where they are at."

Control

Encountering death may bring a sense of losing control as patients experience the inability to halt the dying process. Nurses can take steps to build more control into each day of life for the dying person. Strategies that contribute to a sense of control include the following (Enes, 2003; Tang, 2003; Volker, Kahn, & Penticuff, 2004a; 2004b):

- Protect dignity (privacy, control over body functions, self-care where possible).

- Provide effective management of pain and other symptoms.

- Involve patients in making treatment decisions, including initiation and cessation.

- Encourage determination of how to spend remaining time in ways that acknowledge engagement in living.

- Acknowledge and support patients' desires to manage the financial and emotional effect on family members.

- Provide for place, space, and management of logistics of the dying process.

Additional suggested nursing interventions for enhancing patient control include

- giving bad news in a context of choices,

- managing physical and emotional care to give control over discomfort,

- giving practical information that facilitates navigation of care systems,

- educating to provide knowledge that empowers decision-making, and

- providing a nonthreatening environment that reduces "white-coat" formality (Du Penn & Robison, 2006; Volker, Kahn, & Penticuff, 2004a).

We can empower patients by encouraging them to take responsibility for decisions that affect their quality of life (Poor & Gary, 2001). For some patients, control means receiving active treatment, although they recognize the reality of impending death. Some patients may even view choosing hospice as giving up control (Volker, Kahn, & Penticuff, 2004a; 2004b).

Dignity

As a human characteristic, dignity is shown through respect for self and others (Jacelon, Connelly, Brown, Proulx, & Vo, 2004). A survey of nurses about actions used to promote dignified dying contributed to the following recommended definition of dignified dying: "verbalizes relief of pain, expresses control of symptoms, participates in decisions for care and treatment, verbalizes physical comfort, verbalizes spiritual contentment, and reviews life experiences" (Wilson, Coenen, & Doorenbos, 2006, p. 41). Coenen, Doorenbos, and Wilson (2007) developed the dignity-conserving care model, a holistic approach based on analysis of a dignified dying survey completed by nurses from four countries, including the US.

Three aspects of dignified dying emerged from the study to form the model:

1. attending to symptomatic relief for illness-related concerns,

2. providing a repertoire of psychological and spiritual resources (the importance of specific resources varied between countries), and

3. conducting a social dignity inventory to strengthen environmental resources. Environmental resources included encouraging family members to be present, supporting them, and educating them; respecting privacy boundaries; and respecting and honoring the decisions of patients and families.

"At a basic level, a good death is one that is free from stress and suffering and is consistent with the desires of patients and families."

Nurses who promote patient and family dignity treat each experience as unique and do not judge patient and family values, preferences, lifestyles, or views of life and death (Coyle, 2006).

What Is a Good Death?

Although the term "good death" has different meanings for people (Ciccarello, 2003), many studies and articles report similar components that characterize a good death. At a basic level, a good death is one that is free from stress and suffering and is consistent with the desires of patients and families (Field & Cassell, 1997). Ciccarello (2003) adds that a good death gives one the opportunity to live until death. An analysis of focus groups and in-depth interviews with the many stakeholders involved in end-of-life care and decisions (providers, patients, and family members) resulted in identification of six components of a good death (Steinhauser et al., 2000):

1. Pain and symptom management,

2. Clear decision-making,

3. Preparation for death,

4. Completion (faith issues, life review, resolving conflicts, saying goodbye),

5. Contributing to others, and

6. Affirmation of the whole person.

Other common elements of a good death indicated in the literature include avoiding a prolonged dying process, having a sense of control, strengthening relationships, and not being alone (Center for Bioethics, 2005). For long-term care settings, additional themes of quality end-of-life care that contribute to a good death are creating a homelike environment through providing for privacy and conveniences for family members and having adequate institutional resources of staffing, equipment, and supplies (Brazil et al., 2004). In the intensive care environment, discomfort with death and the existence of a rescue culture may impede the capacity to support a good death (Boyle, Miller, & Forbes-Thompson, 2005).

To facilitate a good death, we can also pay attention to the aesthetic qualities of the dying process—meaning the ways patients see and experience their world. Steeves and Kahn (2006) have adapted the writings of Thomas Aquinas to identify boundaries, rhythm, and clarity as qualities of aesthetic judgment. Defining boundaries has to do with the beginning, middle, and ending experiences of dying. Patients share stories or narratives about their dying experience. They may use metaphors such as going on a journey, passing, moving on, packing a bag, getting on a train, giving up, and letting go to describe their experience.

We can validate these metaphors by listening and by facilitating choices about the place and environment a patient chooses for the ending experience. Patients find their own rhythm in dying. Although we can know the signs and symptoms of death, patients may choose their time based on criteria that we do not always understand. At the end there is clarity of meaning—an understanding and acceptance of the occurrence of death. There is deep sadness, but no regrets for what could have been done. If a patient's narrative is not consistent with a good death, we can offer another perspective or reframe the death experience. We can interpret the narrative in a way that contributes to meaning for a patient, and we can "orchestrate the death" by offering comfort measures and creating an environment of the patient's choice (Steeves & Kahn, 2006).

How to Give Bad News and Support Hope

Although giving information about prognosis is most often in the physician's domain, clinical nurse specialists may also have responsibility for revealing a poor prognosis. All nurses who work with dying patients need to be prepared to respond to the aftermath of bad news, regardless of who delivers the news. Patients and families may be unable to absorb the bad news, they may deny the reality of what they are told, or they may not fully comprehend the message. Patient and family understanding and acceptance can take time. It is the nurse who journeys along with them to support the process of coming to terms with their new reality. As nurses, we are expected to answer questions about prognosis and treatment. Patients identify us as primary sources of information and emotional support, and we are the link between patients and physicians (Barclay, Blackhall, & Tulsky, 2007).

A consensus panel of physicians and patients developed the following guidelines for breaking bad news (Girgis & Sanson-Fisher, 1995):

1. Ensure privacy and adequate time for discussion.

2. Assess patient and family understanding.

3. Provide information about diagnosis and prognosis simply and honestly.

4. Avoid euphemisms and medical jargon.

5. Encourage expression of feelings.

6. Be empathetic.

7. Give a broad, realistic (not overly optimistic) time frame for prognosis.

8. Arrange for follow-up.

Another well-known standard for breaking bad news is the SPIKES Protocol (see sidebar), developed by Baile et al. (2000). As discussed in Chapter 2, patients and families have different desires for information. Individual preferences for disclosure of information must be assessed to tailor the discussion to the ability of patients and families to comprehend and accept the bad news (Ngo-Metzger, August, Srinivasan, Liao, & Meysekens, 2007). Although patients and families generally want a realistic picture of the prognosis, they also want to hear it presented positively (Barclay et al., 2007). Because some patients do not want a full appraisal of their situation, it is always best to ask about what information they do want to hear.

Several researchers have analyzed types of awareness regarding prognosis among dying patients. Open awareness—acknowledgement of the inevitability of death—originally described by Glaser and Strauss in 1968, was further subdivided by Timmerman (1994) into categories of *suspended open awareness* (usually a temporary, early reaction of denial when receiving bad news), *uncertain open awareness* (overlooking negative aspects to focus on hope for a good outcome), and *active open awareness* (accepting the reality of the information and acting based on that reality). Asking the questions "What have you been told about your illness so far?" or "What do you think is happening?" can provide a way to assess unrealistic expectations or denial a patient or family may have (Baile et al., 2000).

SPIKES Protocol

Setting Up: Organize an interview with the patient.

Perception: Find out what the patient knows about his or her illness.

Invitation: Ask if it is OK to give bad news.

Knowledge: Give bad news at level that is understood by the patient.

Emotions: Acknowledge and respond to the patient's emotions.

Strategy and **S**ummary: Summarize what was discussed and determine a follow-up plan.

Source: Baile et al., 2000

Misunderstandings are always a risk with imparting bad news. Statistical terms may not be meaningful, or they may be interpreted to make them sound positive when they are not. Some groups of patients are more likely to misunderstand information about prognosis—in particular, depressed patients, patients with lower levels of education, and men (Barclay et al., 2007). One rule of thumb to use when giving bad news is to limit messages to three facts at a time, and validate accurate understanding before continuing the discussion (Barclay et al.). When giving bad news to patients, an important point for care providers to remember is to avoid phrases that may be misinterpreted by patients and families. See sidebar, "Confusing Messages in Conveying Bad News."

Confusing Messages in Conveying Bad News

"There's nothing we can do for you."

Patients may feel abandoned; instead, focus on ability to control symptoms to help them feel better.

"It's time to think about withdrawal of care."

Patients may perceive this as unsympathetic about what happens to them; instead, suggest it is time to focus on treatment of symptoms. Share that you will stay with them no matter what decision they make.

"Do you want us to do everything that we can to keep you alive?"

Patients may believe they will get inferior care if they say "no"; instead, ask if they want life support or if they have a preference for a more natural death.

"You've failed the treatment."

Patients may interpret this as personal failure; instead, tell them that they are not responding to the treatment in the way that was hoped and ask how they are doing.

"I think you should consider hospice."

Patients may interpret this as hopelessness; instead, tell them they will have coordinated care from a team of professionals who will treat their symptoms and help them stay comfortable.

Source: Ngo-Metzger et al., 2007, p. 172.

Health professional attitudes and behaviors also affect the accuracy and clarity of bad news. Gordon, Buchman, and Buchman (2007) suggest that it is a professional duty to provide truthful information about a patient's prognosis. They also express concern about the occurrence of overly optimistic prognoses, which can lead to misunderstandings. Also, fear and the stress of giving difficult news may contribute to an unclear message. Finding the right balance between honesty and compassion, based on a patient's capacity for understanding and accepting bad news, is indeed challenging. Cultural background is also an important factor to consider when giving bad news, because Western culture emphasizes truth-telling while some cultures believe that verbalizing bad news may be damaging in itself (Gordon et al.).

Some providers worry that patients will lose hope when they are given the truth about their prognosis (Barclay et al., 2007). However, hope can be focused on obtainable goals and outcomes of care, such as symptom control and supportive resources, as patients begin to transition to a shorter life view and think about how to make the best of each day (Johnson, 2007).

"Hope is exactly what is needed to stay engaged in living while shouldering the burden of an uncertain future."

Hope improves quality of life at the end of life. Research has found that hope can be maintained in the terminal phase of illness, and that one begins to focus on "being" rather than "doing." The focus changes to valuing relationships and leaving a legacy (Ersek, 2006). Hope also can be unrealistic and keep patients and families from planning effectively for support during the dying process, although unrealistic hope may also facilitate coping (Johnson, 2007). Back, Arnold, and Quill (2003) suggest an approach that combines hoping for the best while preparing for the worst. An exclusive focus on hope may result in choosing therapies that are more likely to be futile, rather than spending time and energy on improving life quality at the end of life—managing pain and symptoms, addressing fears and concerns, and focusing on relationships. A patient's hopes need to be respected but can also be discussed within the context of the prognosis. While coping through being hopeful, patients can prepare for the worst by being encouraged to complete advance directives and take care of financial and other family matters.

What is hope? Hope is a confident expectation of achieving a future goal, which the person sees as both significant and possible (Dufault & Martocchio, 1985). "Hope is exactly what is needed to stay engaged in living while shouldering the burden of an uncertain future" (Johnson, 2007, p. 451). Johnson conducted a concept analysis of hope based on 17 qualitative studies and found 10 attributes of hope for patients and families as they live with terminal illness. See sidebar, "Attributes of Hope in Terminal Illness." Although patients stated that health professionals sometimes viewed their hope as denial, they also viewed nurses as catalysts for hope.

Nurses can encourage the attributes of hope summarized by Johnson (2007) through focused and supportive communication. Ersek (2006) suggests the following interventions that indicate and support hope for terminally ill patients:

1. Experiential processes that involve sharing stories and enjoying activities.

2. Spiritual processes that can involve spiritual practice and rituals, spiritual counseling, or journaling about experiences.

3. Relational processes with time for emphasizing relationships and building a support system.

4. Rational thought processes that focus on determining goals, finding a sense of control, and identifying what has gone well.

Honest, clear, and caring communication is foundational to each of these categories of hope-fostering interventions.

Attributes of Hope in Terminal Illness

Positive expectations

Tomorrow will be a better day, even when facing a terminal prognosis.

Personal qualities

Inner strength, determination, and optimism promote enjoyment of remaining time and a sense of peace and acceptance.

Spirituality

One does not give up faith and has a purpose for living one's remaining life.

Goals

Goals are short-term and focused on spending high-quality time with family and friends or being involved in a special activity.

Comfort

One is free from pain and comfortable in order to enjoy remaining time.

Help and Caring

Others provide help through encouragement, trust, presence, listening, humor, being honest, and providing information.

Interpersonal Relationships

Relationships with others are loving and honest.

Control

Control is achieved through choices that support autonomy.

Legacy

One leaves behind memories that others will value.

Life Review

One looks back on life and acknowledges positive achievements and contributions to the lives of others.

Source: Johnson, 2007

Life Review

Nurses can use life review to assist dying people in validating their life experiences and accomplishments, healing relationships, and accepting their legacy. "Life review is the systematic and structured process of recalling past events and memories in an effort to find meaning in and achieve resolution in one's life" (Jenko, Gonzalez, & Seymour, 2007, p. 159). Life review is different from reminiscence, which is a more spontaneous recall of memories and often involves storytelling and nostalgia (Haber, 2006). Life review may be structured around specific life themes such as family, work, and major life events and has the potential to result in emotional and relational healing. Through a review of memories and the emotions that accompany the memories, conflicts and old problems may be re-examined. The potential exists for making amends and restoring harmony. A dying person has the opportunity to reframe perceptions of mistakes, failures, or regrets to consider what has been gained from these experiences. Through life review, forgiveness of self and others is possible. Reflection on past lost opportunities can help a person find positive goals for the present (Jenko et al.). Life review is usually evaluative as the person considers how memories contribute to life meaning. It can also be educational or therapeutic (Haber).

"Life review promotes reconciliation through reflecting on one's accomplishments and disappointments with the goal of resolving what is unfinished and moving toward peace about accepting the contributions made to the lives of others."

From a theory perspective, Erikson's (1982) "ego integrity vs. despair" stage of psychosocial development helps us understand the purpose of life review. Life review can result in the perception that one's life has been meaningful (ego integrity). Younger persons with a terminal illness may also experience this later life stage; crisis theory indicates that a terminal illness diagnosis throws them forward to face developmental tasks inconsistent with their chronological age (Trueman & Parker, 2006). "Coming to terms" is another way of understanding life review. Based on an analysis of life review projects, Haber (2006) suggests that adults either come to terms with their past or they do not. They will value the good things in their life; they will either come to terms with the difficult things (major challenges and losses), or they will become obsessed with past failures and conflicts.

Some concerns about using life review include the possibility of negative consequences such as preoccupation, guilt, or despair concerning past experiences (Jenko et al., 2007). In some cases, denial may actually be adaptive coping; in such situations, encouraging life review may actually contribute to distress (Haber, 2006). In an analysis of nearly 100 life reviews, negative outcomes occurred for only 7% of the sample (Haight, 1995). Negative outcomes are more likely among depressed persons (Haber). Life review may result in disclosure of information that either strengthens or negatively affects relationships (Jenko et al.).

Callahan and Kelly (1992) write about life review as a way to discover the need for reconciliation. A need for reconciliation is often accompanied by a feeling that something is unfinished or incomplete. If there is recognition that death will not be peaceful, a person may prolong dying to attempt reconciliation. Finding peace with God or a supreme being, atoning for behavior that was not consistent with one's values and standards, mending broken ties, conveying an apology or gratitude, and being disappointed in tasks not done or missed opportunities are all examples of situations that may be healed through reconciliation. Life review promotes reconciliation through reflecting on one's accomplishments and disappointments with the goal of resolving what is unfinished and moving toward peace and acceptance of contributions made to the lives of others.

Although life review can be organized by an individual, the process is most often enhanced through working with a partner or facilitator (Haber, 2006). For nurses who undertake life reviews with patients, the desired outcome for the patient is a sense of acceptance and integrity of self (Jenko et al., 2007).

Before undertaking a life review process, it is important to manage any need for pain and symptom relief and provide for privacy. Jenko et al. suggest beginning with the question "What part of yourself would you like to leave with the ones who love you?" Other prompts include asking about childhood, family members, and what was important and satisfying in life. As with all communication in working with dying persons, keeping the conversation focused, using open-ended questions, and listening can facilitate the life review process. If a patient is unable or unwilling to participate, you can work with the family to complete a life review; the process can help family members with their grieving process and finding purpose in life (Jenko et al., 2007).

One study involved analysis of the perceptions of 68 community nurses who used life review in palliative care (Trueman & Parker, 2006). In focus group interviews, the community nurses reported both benefits and possible negative effects for patients. Many participants also indicated they were uncertain about the process and wanted more training in life review. Nurses also expressed concern about their own emotional burden resulting from listening to patients, and some said they felt out of their depth and needed supervision. The authors concluded that life review offers a more structured approach for responding to the emotional needs of dying patients. Nurses who wish to use life review can seek additional resources and education on the process. The Hospice Institute of the Florida Suncoast offers a life review toolkit (www.thehospice.org) that can be used as a guide for conducting life reviews.

Art Therapy

Another strategy to assist in cognitive and emotional expression is art therapy. Although art therapy is useful for all ages, it can be particularly useful for children who may not have the verbal skills to talk about their experience. Art therapy can help to express anxiety and loss. Children and others can be encouraged to explain their drawings. Not making assumptions about the meaning of the art is important. Also, provide a psychologically safe environment by limiting any focus on technical skills or creativity. Art therapy can bring to knowledge what has not previously been understood and can enhance self-esteem (Devlin, 2006).

Responding to the Needs of Families

You can help families by providing the information and strategies needed for supporting and comforting their dying family members. By taking actions to help patients and families work toward a peaceful death, nurses will have less stress, feel less helpless, and have less guilt and regret because of attributing difficulties to their own inadequacies (Kristjanson, Hudson, & Oldham, 2003). Families have many needs: They want to know how to provide comfort, how to talk with other family members about the situation, how to manage treatment and side effects, what to expect about changes in a patient's condition, and how to communicate with the patient. They need reassurance, information, and emotional support (Ferrell, Rhiner, Cohen, & Grant, 1991; Kristjanson et al.). Families may not know they have some of these needs—and they may not know how to tell nurses that they have these needs. This requires sensitivity and perceptiveness on your part.

Assessing a patient's important relationships to determine who should be given information is a good way to begin (Dahlin & Giansiracusa, 2006). Understanding a patient's definition of *family* is also important, because their family could include nonrelatives (Zerwekh, 2006). Use a systems perspective to assess family structure, roles, relationships, communication patterns, knowledge deficits, and available resources (Goetschius & Matzo, 2006). Determine whether the family's plan and the patient's plan for end-of-life care are consistent. Assess how well family caregivers are coping with the added responsibilities. They may feel overwhelmed, need relief, have unmet emotional needs, be dealing with family conflicts, and be trying to manage their own and the patient's suffering (Zerwekh). Family members may find the patient's deterioration in mental status to be especially distressing (Ferrell et al., 1991). To assess family coping patterns, Zerwekh suggests asking, "How did your family work things out last time there was a family crisis?" (p. 249). Davies (2006) offers an explanation of the family transition process that you can use to help understand what families are experiencing and what interventions are likely to be needed and effective at what time. See sidebar, "Family Transition Process in Responding to the Death of a Loved One."

Family Transition Process in Responding to the Death of a Loved One

Redefining

Family members need to shift roles and responsibilities to manage the new situation.

Burdening

Patients are concerned about being a burden, while family members adjust to bear the burden.

Struggling With the Paradox

Patients and family members want to maintain a normal life, but also need to face reality and prepare for impending death.

Contending With Change

With a dramatic change and new responsibilities, family members encounter change in many aspects of life, including relationships, roles, and employment.

Searching for Meaning

Family members look for philosophical and spiritual answers to what is happening.

Living Day-to-Day

The patient and family focus on making the most of each day and finding satisfaction in the moment, rather than planning ahead.

Preparing for Death

The patient and family focus on completion of financial and legal tasks, household arrangements, and funeral planning.

Source: Davies, 2006

After assessing how a family is responding to having a dying family member, you can use communication interventions to encourage the family to work through emotions, determine information needs, and manage caregiving challenges. See sidebar, "Interventions to Help Families."

Interventions to Help Families

- With family members, discuss a plan to share information and discuss their concerns to prevent conflict that results from communication mistakes. Provide the family with a notebook and pen to record conversations and write down questions.

- Assist family members in connecting by encouraging them to communicate with one another.

- Explore how to accomplish relationship completion tasks through the following shared messages between family members: Forgive me. I forgive you. I love you. Thank you. Goodbye.

- Explain the normalcy of expressions of feelings and that communication patterns with one another most likely will not change as they respond to the death of a loved one.

- Assist the family in identifying coping strategies, such as taking one day at a time, seeking information to reduce uncertainty, and finding ways to reduce the additional burdens in their lives.

- Discuss what is positive about the caregiving role and convey that many family members have found that caring for a dying relative is rewarding.

- Encourage self-care by discussing ways to meet emotional needs and avoid fatigue and burnout from the caregiving role.

- Provide referral contact information to useful resources.

- Provide information about frequently used medical terms.

- Ensure easy access to health care team; effective communication among health care team members will facilitate meeting the needs of families.

- Identify two contact people, one from the health care organization and the other from the family, who will have the latest information on the patient's condition.

- Use a question and answer sheet for questions from family and responses from health care providers.

- Provide updates on a daily basis.

- Organize a family meeting that includes interdisciplinary health team members. Discuss and rehearse the roles of interdisciplinary team members before a family conference.

- Consider using a speaker phone for family members who are not able to be physically present.

- If family members are unable to talk to one another, you might find it necessary to act as an intermediary in communicating information and decisions.

Sources: Boyle et al., 2005; Byock, 1997; Davies, 2006; Ferrell et al., 1991; Royak-Schaler et al., 2006; Zerwekh, 2006

Several models and research studies exist concerning the use of family meetings for planning end-of-life care. King and Quill (2006) suggest a family relational model to guide interactions with families. The model uses a family systems interpretive approach as opposed to the more traditional individualistic approach with emphasis on patient autonomy. Families have different levels of relational ability. Families with healthy relationships and strong bonds will have the ability to move on quickly to shared problem solving and arrive at a consensus about end-of-life care decisions.

Some families may have difficulty talking about emotionally intense subjects. If they close off discussion about a terminal prognosis, using the approach of hoping for the best, but preparing for the worst may help them to move forward on decision-making. However, some families have a troubling relational history and will not communicate or collaborate well. For families whose communication shows disorganization, conflict, hostility, or lack of commitment, the health care team will need to spend more time in planning and use a higher level of structure in family meetings to decrease conflict, and will likely need to debrief following the family meeting (King & Quill, 2006). The Checklist of Family Relational Abilities (see Appendix B) is a clinical tool that can be used by health care team members to assess families from a family systems perspective.

Family meetings will be more effective if they are early, proactive, and scheduled for anyone who is at a significant risk for death (Boyle et al., 2005). Holding a family meeting will provide health care team members with the following opportunities: a time set aside to discuss the patient's situation honestly and sensitively, knowledge about patient and family views and preferences, identification of families who may have high conflict or difficulty understanding the situation, and achievement of consensus on care strategies. Scheduling an interdisciplinary pre-conference before the family meeting can ensure that consistent information will be provided. The following recommended format offers an effective structure for implementing a family meeting:

- Begin with introductions.

- State the goals of the meeting.

- Ask what the patient and family understand about the medical diagnosis.

- Assess fears and worries.

- Determine how much information is wanted.

- Identify any other persons the patient would like to have involved.

- Invite or prompt the patient or family to talk if either is quiet.

- Act as a translator for medical terminology if needed (Dahlin & Gianiracusa, 2006).

An analysis of audiotapes of 51 interdisciplinary family conferences (physicians, social workers, nurses, and chaplains) indicated missed opportunities for effective communication in 29% of the conferences (Curtis et al., 2005). Examples of missed opportunities were

- not answering a question,

- answering a different question than what was asked,

- a lack of acknowledging emotions when words such as "sad" were used, and

- not exploring family comments about treatment preferences.

Family members expressed greater satisfaction with communication when health care providers spent more time listening than talking. Another study showed how nonabandonment of patient and family was expressed in family conferences in the intensive care setting (West, Engelbergh, Wenrich, & Curtis, 2005).

Actions that communicated nonabandonment from professionals were direct reassurance, assurance of comfort, accessibility, and expressions of valuing the family. Families also expressed their concern about possible abandonment by professionals and not wanting to abandon their dying family member. They asked directly about being abandoned by professionals, asked clinicians to honor the patient's wishes, asked for protection from suffering, requested to be present at the time of death, and acknowledged their readiness to "let go" and wanting professionals to concur with them in that decision.

Jones (2007) conducted a randomized control trial to compare a proactive family conference with the standard family-staff interactions and usual conference strategy. The proactive strategy included a bereavement brochure and had five specific objectives:

1. Valuing and appreciating what family members had to say.

2. Acknowledging their emotions.

3. Listening (more than talking).

4. Asking questions to get a better sense of who the patient is as a person.

5. Encouraging family members to ask questions.

The proactive strategy resulted in fewer symptoms of post-traumatic stress disorder, anxiety, and depression when the two groups were compared 90 days after the death of a patient. Models and evidence-based strategies for family meetings can guide health care teams in planning meetings that will respond to the needs of family members. Preparation, adequate time, and good communication among professionals are also needed to implement suggested strategies.

Reflective Practice

At the end of life, patients and their families have unique needs and will express them in unique ways. The sensitivity and listening that are a part of nursing presence (*see* Chapter 1) are useful tools for learning to read the cues that patients and family members give us. Verbal capacity certainly facilitates the process for understanding needs. However, culture, family dynamics, a reluctance to be vulnerable, and the expectation to remain strong and independent can all interfere with asking for what is needed. And so we must be cautious and identify assumptions that we hold about what patients and families need.

In caring for patients at the end of life, we may experience tension between promoting patient autonomy and listening to the family as a unit, especially when the family may not be unified in their understanding and approach toward supporting their dying family member. In American culture, we often consider the needs of the individual over the needs of the group. This mind-set may lead us to put patients first and value family members' perspectives less. Although it is not intentional, our culture leads us in this direction.

Norwegians are led by their culture as well, but with differing perspectives. Interviews with health professionals in Norway consistently conveyed the message that family is important. In their cultural thinking, the family remains after their loved one is gone, so Norwegian health professionals wanted the family members to know that everything possible was done for their dying family member, so they would have no regrets after the death. The Norwegian health professionals did not mean that all technology should be used to try to keep life going when it was futile. Instead, they often made decisions about the most appropriate medical care, given the patient's situation, and interpreted what should be done based on their assessment. However, if a family member insisted on life-prolonging treatment (such as transfer from a nursing home to a hospital) and the family member could not be persuaded to follow the health professional's recommendation, Norwegian health professionals would do what the family members wanted for the benefit of the family, as they would go on living with the consequences of their decisions after the death.

Because we bring our own experiences and beliefs to the bedside, it is good to step back and ask ourselves some questions before caring for our dying patients:

- How do I define hope at the end of life?

- Does my definition differ from the patient and family?

- How do I define a good death?

Ethical Practice in Responding to Family Wishes

ETHICAL PROBLEM: What should I do if families insist that we continue IV fluids, when the patient will likely be more comfortable without them?

What should I value?

- Comfort of the patient.
- Peace of mind for family members.
- Effective use of health care resources.
- Facilitating a good death.

Who should I be?

- Compassionate.
- An advocate for the patient's comfort as well as an advocate for meeting the needs of the family.
- A competent nurse who uses best practices in end-of-life care.

What should I do?

- Work with health care team to develop a unified approach to explaining the effects of IV fluids at this stage of care.
- Explore fears and concerns family members have about discontinuing IV fluids.
- Educate about advantages and disadvantages of IV fluids for patients.
- Consider discussion of a time-limited trial with re-evaluation at an agreed upon time-frame.
- Assure them that you will support their decision.

Nurses' Stories

Hope and Control

Patients and families don't always make the decisions we would like for them to make. As a hospital clinical nurse specialist said, "We often have our own agenda."

I was taking care of this woman in her 40s with ovarian cancer. She was in and out of our oncology unit many times. The doctors kept saying, "Go home and get your affairs in order." But she kept coming back for more treatment. I knew she would be more comfortable and have a better quality of life if she stopped treatment, but I respected her decision. The bottom line is that people don't want to be dead! I learned from her how hard it is to accept that you are dying. She wanted to live and that was her hope.

Autonomy and Self-Determination

In a medical system that follows the principle of individual autonomy, sometimes we struggle when working with cultures and systems that focus more on family than individuals. A hospice nursing supervisor told of the controversy the interdisciplinary team had to work through when a family did not allow the patient to be told about hospice or to sign the consent form.

I was supervising a hospice program when we got a referral for an elderly Southeast Asian immigrant. The children requested that we not talk with him about dying. Staff members were in a quandary, because we require a signed consent to [begin] hospice. As we discussed it in our interdisciplinary team meeting, we decided that the family could be proxy for the consent, because individual autonomy was not a cultural norm for them. We cared for the patient throughout his end-of-life journey without using the word "hospice" or discussing dying with him. When he died, the family thanked us for our care.

Delivering Bad News

Often, nurses are the ones who have to follow up after bad news is delivered. The importance of presence and compassion cannot be overemphasized. A hospice nurse told about her personal experience.

I think one of the reasons I got into hospice was a negative experience that I had at my child's death. She was 2 days old, and I distinctly remember that the only thing a nurse said to me was, "Will you sign the autopsy form?" And I think there are no right words to say, but I think a nurse's presence and just saying, "I'm so sorry" rather than running in and out of the room are so helpful. "I'm sorry" would have helped.

Key Points

- Elicit patients and families' perspectives. Ask open-ended questions such as, "What is your understanding of the illness?" "What do you think is happening?" "What do you want to happen?"

- Understand that hope is subjective and can be defined in many ways. Again, ask open-ended questions such as, "What do you hope for (today, next week, next month)?

- Autonomy and control are important to patients and families. Families need to be included in decision-making. However, individual autonomy is not necessarily a value in all cultures. Cultural sensitivity includes asking about decision-making.

- Delivering bad news involves assessment of patients and families' understanding, clear and compassionate communication, and careful listening.

REFLECTION QUESTIONS

1. What does a good death mean to you? What are some examples of how patients and family members might have different meanings of a good death?

2. What strategies will you use to respond to a patient who is upset, angry, or discouraged about receiving bad news?

3. How can you balance helping patients and families understand the reality of their diagnosis and prognosis with their need to have hope?

References

Back, A. L., Arnold, R. M., & Quill, T. E. (2003). Hope for the best, and prepare for the worst. *Annals of Internal Medicine, 138*(5), 439-443.

Baile, W. F., Buckman, R., Lenzi, R., Glober, G., Beale, E. A., & Kudelka, A.P. (2000). SPIKES: A six-step protocol for delivering bad news: Application to the patient with cancer. *The Oncologist, 5*(4), 302-311.

Barclay, J. S., Blackhall, L. J., & Tulsky, J. A. (2007). Communication strategies and cultural issues in the delivery of bad news. *Journal of Palliative Medicine, 10*(4), 958-977.

Boyle, D. K., Miller, P. A., & Forbes-Thompson, S. A. (2005). Communication and end-of-life care in the intensive care unit: Patient, family, and clinician outcomes. *Critical Care Nursing Quarterly, 28*(4), 3-2-316.

Brazil, K., McAiney, C., Caron-O'Brien, M., Kelley, M. L., O'Krafka, P., & Sturdy-Smithy, C. (2004). Quality end-of-life care in long-term care facilities: Service providers' perspectives. *Journal of Palliative Care,20*(2), 85-92.

Byock, I. (1997). *Dying Well: The prospects for growth at the end of life.* New York: Riverhead Books.

Callahan, M., & Kelley, P. (1992). *Final gifts: Understanding the special awareness, needs, and communications of the dying.* New York: Bantam.

Center for Bioethics. (2005). *End of life care: An ethical overview.* University of Minnesota. Retrieved March 21, 2008, from http://www.ahc.umn.edu/bioethics/publications/bioethics_overviews.html

Ciccarello, G. P. (2003). Strategies to improve end-of-life care in the intensive care unit. *Dimensions of Critical Care Nursing, 22*(5), 216-222.

Coenen, A., Doorenbos, A. Z., & Wilson, S. A. (2007). Nursing interventions to promote dignified dying in four countries. *Oncology Nursing Forum, 34*(6), 1151-1156.

Coyle, N. (2006). Introduction to palliative nursing care. *Textbook of palliative nursing* (pp. 5-46). New York: Oxford University Press.

Curtis, J. R., Engelberg, R. A., Wenrich, M. D., Shannon, S. E., Treece, P. D., & Rubenfeld, G. D. (2005). Missed opportunities during family conferences about end-of-life care in the intensive care unit. *American Journal of Respiratory Critical Care Medicine,171*, 844-849.

Dahlin, C. M., & Gianiracusa, D. E. Communication in palliative care. (2006). In B. R. Ferrell & N. Coyle (Eds.), *Textbook of palliative nursing* (pp. 67-93). New York: Oxford University Press.

Davies, B. (2006). Supporting families in palliative care. In B. Ferrell & N. Coyle (Eds.), *Textbook of palliative nursing* (pp. 545-560). New York: Oxford University Press.

Devlin, B. (2006). The art of healing and knowing in cancer and palliative care. *International Journal of Palliative Nursing, 12*(1), 16-19.

Dufault, K., & Martocchilo, B. (1985). Hope: Its spheres and dimensions. *Nursing Clinics of North America, 20*, 379-391.

Du Penn, A. R., & Robison, J. (2006). The outpatient setting. In B. R. Ferrell & N. Coyle (Eds.), *Textbook of palliative nursing* (pp. 835-845). New York: Oxford University Press.

Enes, S. P. (2003). An exploration of dignity in palliative care. *Palliative Medicine, 17*, 263-269.

Erikson, E. H. (1982). *The life cycle completed: A review.* New York: Norton.

Ersek, M. (2006). The meaning of hope in the dying. In B. R. Ferrell & N. Coyle (Eds.), *Textbook of palliative nursing* (pp. 513-529). New York: Oxford University Press.

Ferrell, B. R., Rhiner, M., Cohen, M., & Grant, M. (1991). Pain as a metaphor for illness. Part I: Impact of pain on family caregivers. *Oncology Nursing Forum, 22*(8), 1303-9.

Field, M. J., & Cassell, C. K. (1997). *Approaching death: Improving care at the end of life.* Washington, D.C.: National Academy Press.

Girgis, A., & Sanson-Fisher, R. W. (1995). Breaking bad news: Consensus guidelines for medical practitioners. *Journal of Clinical Oncology, 13,* 2449-2456.

Glaser, B., & Strauss, A. (1968). *Awareness of Dying.* Chicago: Aldine.

Goetschius, S. K., & Matzo, M. L. (2006).Caring for families: The other patient in palliative care. In M. L. Matzo & D. W. Sherman (Eds.), *Palliative care nursing* (pp. 247-272). New York: Springer Publishing.

Gordon, M., Buchman, D., & Buchman, S. H. (2007). "Bad news' communication in palliative care: A challenge and key to success. *Annals of Long-Term Care, 15*(4), 32-38.

Haber, D. (2006). Life review: Implementation, theory, research, and therapy. The *International Journal of Aging and Human Development, 63*(2), 153-171.

Haight, B. (1995). Reminiscing: The state of the art as a basis for practice. In J. Hendricks (Ed.), *The meaning of reminiscence and life review* (pp. 21-52). Amityville, NY: Baywood.

Jacelon, C. S., Connelly, T. W., Brown, R., Proulx, K., & Vo, T. (2004). A concept analysis of dignity for older adults. *Journal of Advanced Nursing, 48,* 76-83.

Jenko, M., Gonzalez, L., & Seymour, M. J. (2007). Life review with the terminally ill. *Journal of Hospice and Palliative Nursing, 9*(3), 159-167.

Johnson, S. (2007). Hope in terminal illnes: An evolutionary concept analysis. *International Journal of Palliative Nursing, 13*(9), 451-459.

Jones, T. (2007). A proactive communication strategy reduced post-traumatic stress disorder symptoms in relatives of patients dying in the ICU. *Evidence-Based Nursing, 10*(3), 85.

Kelner, M. (1995). Activists and delegators: Elderly patients' preferences about control at the end of life. *Social Science and Medicine, 41*(4), 537-545.

King, D. A., & Quill, T. (2006). Working with families in palliative care: One size does not fit all. *Journal of Palliative Medicine, 9*(3), 704-715.

Kristjanson, L., Hudson, P., & Oldham, L. (2003). In M. O'Connor. & S. Aranda (Eds.), *Palliative care nursing: A guide to practice* (pp. 272-283). Melbourne: Ausmed.

Ladd, R. E., Pasquella, L., & Smith, S. (2000). What to do when the end is near: Ethical issues in home care nursing. *Public Health Nursing, 17* (2), 103-110.

Ngo-Metzger, Q., August, K. J., Srinivasan, M., Liao, S., & Meysekens, F. L. (2007). End-of-life care: Guidelines for patient-centered communication. *American Family Physician, 77*(2), 167-174.

Poor, B., & Gary, E. (2001). Communicating with the dying patient. In B. Poor & G. P. Poirrier, (Eds.), *End of life nursing care.* (pp.213-235). Sudbury, MA: Jones and Bartlett.

Royak-Schaler, R., Gadalla, S. M., Lemkau, J. P., Roos, D. D., Alexander, C., & Scott, D. (2006). Family perspectives on communication with health care providers during end-of-life cancer care. *Oncology Nursing Forum, 33*(4), 753-760.

Steeves, R., & Kahn, D. (2006). Understanding a good death: James's story. In B. R. Ferrell & N. Coyle (Eds.), *Textbook of palliative nursing* (pp. 1209-1215). New York: Oxford University Press.

Steinhauser, K. E., Clipp, E. C., McNeilly, M., Christakis, N., McIntryre, L. M., & Tulsky, J. A. (2000). In search of a good death: Observations of patients, families, and providers. *Annals of Internal Medicine, 12*(10), 825-832.

Tang, S. T. (2003). When death is imminent: Where terminally ill patients with cancer prefer to die and why. *Cancer Nursing, 26,* 245-251.

Tilden, V. P. (1999). Ethics perspectives on end-of-life care. *Nursing Outlook, 47*(4), 162-167.

Timmerman, S. (1994). Dying of awareness: The theory of awareness contexts revisited. *Social Health Illness, 16*(3), 322-339.

Trueman, I., & Parker, J. (2006). Exploring community nurses' perceptions of life review in palliative care. *Journal of Clinical Nursing, 15,* 197-207.

Volker, D. L., Kahn, D., & Penticuff, J. H. (2004a). Patient control and end-of-life care. Part I: The advanced practice nurse perspective. *Oncology Nursing Forum, 31*(5), 945-953.

Volker, D. L., Kahn, D., & Penticuff, J. H. (2004b). Patient control and end-of-life care. Part II: The patient perspective. *Oncology Nursing Forum, 31*(5), 954-960.

West, H. F., Engelbergh, R. A., Wenrich, M. D., & Curtis, J. R. (2005). Expressions of nonabandonment during the intensive care unit family conference. *Journal of Palliative Medicine, 8*(4), 797-807.

Wilson, S. A., Coenen, A., & Doorenbos, A. (2006). Dignified dying as a nursing phenomenon in the United States. *Journal of Hospice and Palliative Nursing, 8*(1), 34-41.

Zerwekh, J. V. (2006). *Nursing care at the end of life.* Philadelphia: F. A. Davis.

When he was terminal, he just wanted to pray.
That's what he wanted. He asked for painkillers.
He just wanted us to hold his hands and pray with
him. That's what he wanted.

—Norwegian long-term care nurse

4

•

Understanding the Spiritual Journey

At the end of life, spiritual needs of a patient can transcend physical needs. While it is easy to get caught up in the medical aspects of care, unmet spiritual needs can contribute to pain and suffering and should be addressed in the same way we address physical symptoms.

In this chapter, we provide definitions of spirituality and religion, explore spiritual needs, identify barriers in providing spiritual care, and suggest communication strategies to use in supporting patients in their spiritual journeys. In addition, we will discuss the role nurses play in a patient's spiritual journey and strategies for developing competence in spiritual care.

Definitions of Spirituality and Religion

Spirituality is most broadly defined as the quest for meaning and purpose in life, while religion provides a means to express spirituality (Puchalski, Dorff, & Hendi, 2004). While the spirit is part of our being, religion is viewed as a structured belief system that provides a philosophy and ethical code for living (Chochinov & Cann, 2005). This structured belief system often involves the practice of rituals and activities such as reading a holy book, praying, or using liturgy in a community of people who express similar beliefs (Cornette, 2005). Religion can also be viewed as a component of spirituality as conceptualized by the five "R's" of spirituality: reason, reflection, religion, relationships, and restoration (Zerwekh, 2006). As an expression of spirituality, religious beliefs help dying persons make sense of the suffering and uncertainty they experience (Puchalski et al., 2004). Sheldon (2000) describes spiritual journey as a search for the purpose for which one has been created, a private process of self-discovery, and a source of strength that transcends a weak and deteriorating body.

The 5 Rs of Spirituality

1. **Reason**

   Searching for meaning and purpose; finding the will to live.

2. **Reflection**

   Thinking about one's existence; facilitated through art, music, or literature.

3. **Religion**

   Expression of spirituality in institutionalized or informal format; a framework of values and beliefs; involves rituals, religious practices, and reading of sacred texts.

4. **Relationships**

   Connection with others and a deity or higher being; experiences of service, trust, hope, and love.

5. **Restoration**

   Positive influence on health and well-being.

   Source: Zerwekh, 2006, p. 216.

In a review of spirituality literature, Chochinov and Cann (2005) found the following themes that describe various views of spirituality:

- Relationship to God, a spiritual being, a higher power, or a reality greater than self.

- Not of the self.

- Transcendence or connectedness.

- Existential, meaning not of the material world.

- Meaning and purpose in life.

- Life force or personal integration.

From a religious point of view, spirituality involves a sense of connectedness to a personal God, which results in significance and meaning. From a secular perspective, spirituality also provides significance and meaning (Murray, 2004). Spiritual experiences of hope, meaning, reconciliation, and transcendence (Zerwekh, 2006) are relevant at the end of life for both religious and nonreligious persons.

Spiritual Needs

Spirituality is viewed as a universal experience; all humans are presumed to have spiritual needs (Hermann, 2007; Smith, 2006). A majority of the population of the Western world believes in God (95%), and 85% of people worldwide view themselves as religious (Kemp, 2006; Anandarajah & Hight, 2001).

From a nursing perspective, a person's spirituality can be viewed as an innate human characteristic that influences the physiological, psychological, sociocultural, and developmental aspects of a person (Beckman, Baxley-Harges, Bruick-Sorge, & Salmon, 2007). O'Brien (2003) suggests that dying persons have the following universal spiritual needs:

- freedom from loneliness and isolation,

- the opportunity to feel useful,

- the opportunity to express anger and reduce depression,

- comfort in times of anxiety and fear, and

- meaning in the current experience of living and dying.

Other important spiritual needs for dying persons include

* maintaining a sense of self-worth;

* retaining an active role with family and friends;

* leaving a legacy;

* the experience of forgiveness, hope, and love;

* opportunities for religious practices such as prayer and participation in religious services; and

* the need to change what is causing suffering or unhappiness.

(Gauthier, 2002; Hermann, 2007; Kemp, 2006; Murray, 2004; O'Brien, 2003; Ryan, 1997; Taylor, 2006).

Spiritual Pain, Distress, and Suffering

Dying persons may exhibit spiritual pain through expressions of meaninglessness, worthlessness, loneliness, or emptiness (Murata, 2003). Spiritual distress may be indicated by expressions of unresolved anger, guilt, blame, and hatred; absence of joy in life; avoidance of family and friends; and inability to experience comfort in religious participation that previously provided succor (Zerwekh, 2006). Conflict between beliefs and what occurs in life circumstances can be a source of spiritual distress (Anandarajah & Hight, 2001). Suffering is defined as a situation of severe distress that threatens personhood (Cassell, 1991); suffering may be physical, emotional, social, or spiritual (Puchalski et al., 2004). Threats to personal wholeness encountered at the end of life—an unfavorable prognosis, loss of the ability to function, loss of privacy and autonomy, uncontrolled pain, lengthy and recurrent disease, and awareness of one's mortality—all contribute to suffering (Sherman, 2006). The anguish of suffering can be alleviated through understanding the suffering as an opportunity for personal transformation that leads to redemptive relationships with God and others. Ascribing meaning to the suffering helps dying persons and family members to make sense of their experience and cope with threats to their personal wholeness.

"Ascribing meaning to the suffering helps dying persons and family members to make sense of their experience and cope with threats to personal wholeness."

Healing While Dying

Although healing of the body might not be achieved, psychological and spiritual healing is possible in all stages of the life cycle. Gauthier (2002) explains what healing while dying means:

> *The concept of healing within dying allows the person to move beyond the ideas of life and death and to become who she or he has always been, the self that preceded birth and will survive death. The recognition that healing never ends can make a person's life whole. (p. 221)*

In a study of 14 terminally ill adults on healing at the end of life, participants identified that maintaining relationships, having a sense of home, and returning to spiritual roots facilitated healing. They needed to work through barriers to healing such as coping with physical symptoms, relinquishing past roles, and having little time to complete tasks that were important to them. For these participants, healing near the end of life meant experiencing a sense of peace and freedom and feeling accepted and understood (Gauthier, 2002). In healing, dying people can find peace and reconciliation with God, self, and others; can let go of the need to hold onto life; and can move toward a peaceful death (Puchalski et al., 2004).

One definition of healing is restoration to spiritual wholeness (Sherman, 2006). Three tasks can lead people who are dying to spiritual wholeness: finding meaning in life, dying in a way that is true to one's identity, and finding hope beyond the grave (Doka, 1993). In a meta-summary of qualitative research—11 articles with data from 217 adults—Williams (2006) concluded that spiritual work at the end of life leads to spiritual well-being. Characteristics or conditions that contribute to the ability to do spiritual work and healing are:

- the need for a positive outlook;
- the need for involvement and control;

- the need to "finish business";

- the need for hope, goals, and ambitions;

- the need to retain social life and place in community;

- the need to cope with and share emotions; and

- the ability to communicate truthfully and honestly.

Although cure of illness may not be possible, growth at the end of life is possible. An adaptation of Maslow's hierarchy of needs by Zalenski and Raspa (2006) is a framework for understanding how dying people can reach their maximum human potential (see "Hierarchy of Needs for Dying People" sidebar). At the highest level, a dying person reaches transcendence. What does transcendence mean? It is a highly abstract concept that has to do with the mystery of life that is beyond human understanding. Transcendence moves you beyond the limitations of self and death (Kemp, 2006). The dying often go through a detachment and separation from the experienced life that support moving forward to a new reality beyond self and what has been known. A "nearing death awareness" may occur in which you see another world (Zerwekh, 2006). Doing spiritual work can lead to transcendence. Maslow explained that "transcendence is connection to others, the universe, or divinity leading to an intensification of life, a feeling of limitless possibilities, and a sense of wonder and awe" (Zalenski & Raspa, 2006, p. 1123). In a study of the role of spirituality and religion for parents of dying children, transcendence was represented by the parents' belief in the continuation and transformation of the parent-child relationship beyond death (Robinson, Thiel, Backus, & Meyer, 2006). Although nurses cannot make transcendence occur, they can listen to patients' stories of transcendence and witness what cannot be explained (Zerwekh).

Hierarchy of Needs for Dying People

Level 1

Relief of distressing physical symptoms, including pain.

Level 2

Reduction of fears of physical harm, dying, or abandonment.

Level 3

Affection, love, and acceptance through terminal illness experience; mobilization of support systems.

Level 4

Esteem, respect, appreciation, and recognition of contributions.

Level 5

Self-actualization and transcendence.

Source: Zalenski & Raspa, 2006

Why Nurses Do Not Provide Spiritual Care

Reasons for not offering spiritual care or doing a spiritual assessment often have to do with feelings of discomfort and insecurity about using spiritual interventions. You might view spirituality as too sacred and intimate for nursing interventions, and you might believe that spiritual care is the role of the chaplain or a spiritual counselor. A lack of connection with your own spirituality also can lead to discomfort when focusing on the spiritual needs of dying patients and their families (O'Brien, 2003; Sheldon, 2000). You and physician colleagues also may lack education to prepare yourselves to provide spiritual care. Although most patients consider themselves to be spiritual and pray about their health (71% and 75%, respectively, in a study of spiritual concerns of seriously ill patients), many also believed that addressing spiritual concerns was not the role of primary care physicians (Holmes, Rabow, & Dibble, 2006). Patients' views of both nurses and physicians often reflect a dichotomy between the body and mind-spirit that is predominant in Western health care. Patients themselves can become a barrier to spiritual interventions based on their limited role expectations. They may be reluctant to share their spiritual distress with health care providers and might view nurses as being too busy to respond to spiritual concerns (Murray, 2004). In addition, health care system leaders who focus on managed care might not prioritize strategies that promote the spiritual care of dying patients (Sheldon).

Spiritual Standards of Practice

Nurses may lack education and may be uncomfortable with how to provide spiritual care but, nevertheless, providing spiritual care is a practice standard. The Joint Commission on Accreditation of Healthcare Organizations, the American Association of Colleges of Nursing, and the National Council of State Boards of Nursing have all established standards that address providing spiritual care (McEwan, 2005). Although agreement on the definition of spirituality has not emerged, the North American Nursing Diagnosis Association (NANDA) has six diagnostic categories—pulled together from the above-noted organizations' standards—related to spirituality and religion:

- spiritual distress,

- risk for spiritual distress,

- readiness for enhanced spiritual well-being,

- impaired religiosity,

- risk for impaired religiosity, and

- readiness for enhanced religiosity (Sessanna, Finnell, & Jezewski, 2007).

Intervention categories for spiritual care included in the Nursing Outcomes Classification (NOC) are religious ritual enhancement, spiritual support, spiritual growth facilitation, and forgiveness facilitation.

Spiritual Assessment: Beginning the Conversation

A spiritual assessment is a way to open a conversation about the place of spirituality and religion in a patient's life. When patients are unsure or reluctant to make their spiritual needs known, a spiritual assessment can give them "permission" to discuss their spiritual needs (Zerwekh, 2006). The literature includes a variety of questions and assessment tools to identify the spiritual needs of dying persons. Taylor (2006) suggests the use of two questions when a lack of time does not allow a more complete spiritual assessment:

- How does your spirituality help you to live with your illness?

- What can I do to support your spiritual beliefs and practices?

Spiritual Assessment Questions

- What matters the most to you in life?
- What is your source of strength and hope?
- To whom do you turn when you need help?
- What brings you joy and comfort?
- What are you afraid of right now?
- What are your worries?
- What spiritual or religious practices bring you comfort?
- Are there religious books or materials that you want nearby?
- How has your illness changed your view of life?
- What is your greatest wish or hope at this stage of your life?
- How are your spirits?
- Tell me about your spiritual journey.
- What nourishes your spirit?
- How do your beliefs influence the ways you are coping with dying?
- How do your beliefs influence the ways you are making end-of-life decisions?

O'Connor, 1993; Hudson & Rumbold, 2003, p. 77; Sheldon, 2000, p. 9; Zerwekh, 2006, p. 231.

Relevant spiritual assessment questions are focused on the place of God and prayer in a patient's life, one's attitude toward self, quality of relationships with family and friends, and attitude toward religion (Van der Poel, 1998). Stoll (1979) suggested organizing a spiritual assessment by asking about patients' ideas of God or a deity, their sources of hope and strength, their religious practices, and the relationships between their spiritual beliefs and health. Underlying spiritual needs can also be used to guide a nurse's approach to assessment: the need to love and be loved, the need to forgive and experience forgiveness, and the need to find meaning and purpose in life and have hope for the future (Shelly, 2000). Specific spiritual assessment guidelines include SPIRIT, HOPE, FICA, and the Spiritual Needs Inventory. (See sidebar).

Spiritual Assessment Guidelines and Tools

SPIRIT (Highfield, 2000)

S = Spiritual belief system (religious affiliation)

P = Personal spirituality (beliefs and practices)

I = Integration with a spiritual community

R = Ritualized practices and restrictions

I = Implications for medical care

T = Terminal events planning (advance directives, clergy)

HOPE (Cavendish et al., 2007)

H = Sources of hope, meaning, strength, peace, love, and connection

O = Organized religion

P = Personal spiritual and religious practices

E = Effects on medical care and end-of-life issues

FICA (Puchalski, 1999)

F = Faith or beliefs

- What is your faith or belief?

- Do you consider yourself spiritual or religious?

- What things do you believe in that give meaning to your life?

I = Importance and influence

- What influence does faith have on how you take care of yourself?
- How have your beliefs influenced your behavior during this illness?
- What role do your beliefs play in regaining your health?

C = Community

- Are you part of a spiritual or religious community?
- Is this a support to you? How?
- Is there a person or group of people you really love or who are very important to you?

A = Address

- How would you like me, your health care provider, to address these issues in your health care?

Spiritual Needs Inventory (Hermann, 2006)

- Tool is specific to the spiritual needs of dying patients
- Development—qualitative study of 19 hospice patients
- Tested on 100 hospice patients
- 17 items
- Five subscales—outlook, inspiration, spiritual activities, religion, community
- Internal consistency reliability is .85

When conducting a spiritual assessment, we need to respect patients' beliefs and avoid imposing our own religious and spiritual beliefs (Puchalski, 1999). Because spirituality is integrated into our very being, it is important to examine how we use our own spirituality in our work with patients and families. The way we live through our spirituality may be valuable and helpful to our patients, may contribute to discomfort, or may be viewed as intrusive. Before beginning a spiritual assessment, explain why you are asking questions about spirituality and religion. Let patients know that they can share their spiritual beliefs and needs if they feel comfortable with doing so. Listen to the words used by patients and family members that show comfort or lack of comfort with spiritual or religious language (Sherman, 2006).

Children are less likely than adults to be offended by questions about spirituality and religion (Taylor, 2006). To assess religious practices, you can ask, "What do you do before you go to sleep?" or "What do you do on Sunday?" A question for children older than 6 is, "If you could get God to answer one question, what one question would you ask God?" (Sexson, 2004). Conversations with parents are another source of information about the child's spiritual needs. Play and artwork may also provide situations for spiritual assessment of children (Taylor).

Spiritual Interventions

Spiritual care is "meeting people where they are and assisting them in connecting or reconnecting to things, practices, ideas, and principles that are at their core of their being—the breath of their life, making a connection between yourself and that person" (Lunn, 2003, p. 154). Unlike physical-care protocols, spiritual interventions are likely to be more varied and more dependent on the uniqueness of each patient as well as the uniqueness of the nurse. Because spirituality involves the whole person and permeates aspects of physical and psychosocial well-being, a variety of interventions can be used to respond to the spiritual needs of patients and their families. Hudson and Rumbold (2003) suggest that the spiritual care given by one nurse will not be exactly what is given by another nurse. Also, spiritual care is not always a separate set of interventions; acts of care are often experienced as a response to spiritual needs (Hudson & Rumbold). In a study on spiritual interventions used by nurses, many implemented the following interventions to respond to patients' spiritual needs:

1. holding a patient's hand,

2. listening,

3. laughing,

4. praying, and

5. being present (Grant, 2004).

Of these five interventions, only prayer seems overtly spiritual or religious. Sheldon (2000) suggests that as a nurse, you must first understand your own spirituality in order to understand the spirituality of another. One strategy that may seem nonthreatening in the realm of spiritual interventions for both patient and nurse is a communication strategy called "WEB," suggested by Mathews (Sherman, 2006) for connecting with patients about their spirituality:

- **W** refers to welcoming patients by showing acceptance and letting them know they are free to talk about what is important to them.

- **E** is providing encouragement through acknowledging the importance of spiritual and religious practices—ask patients what would be helpful to them.

- **B** means expressing blessings in a way that is sensitive to a patient's faith tradition—blessings to you, God bless you, shalom, and so on.

Spiritual Interventions in Nursing Care

- Touch the patient.

- Relieve physical symptoms, allowing the patient to focus on meeting spiritual needs.

- Help patients participate in religious rituals of their choice; facilitate needs that cannot be met independently, such as locating televised or recorded religious services.

- Provide quiet time for prayer; encourage and offer prayer that is consistent with a patient's beliefs.

- Provide an opportunity for spiritual concerns to emerge.

- Refer patients to religious practitioners when a desire to do so is indicated; consult with a chaplain or religious counselor about ways to meet spiritual needs of a patient.

- Review and reaffirm a patient's circumstances, beliefs, and relationships.

- Provide opportunity for a patient to reflect on successes and failures, hopes, fears, grief, and sorrow.

- Promote spiritual integration by identifying ways to assist patients in completing unfinished business and repairing broken relationships.

- Encourage families to provide symbols of the faith traditions of patients.
- Arrange to provide religious reading materials, music, and worship that give spiritual support to patients.
- Mobilize support from family, church members, and community.
- Assign nurses who have expertise in spiritual care to patients who have greater spiritual needs.
- Set realistic goals for last days.
- Explore with patients the need and desire for forgiveness in relationships.

Hermann, 2007; Hudson & Rumbold, 2003; Kemp, 2006; Mickley & Cowles, 2001; O'Gorman, 2002; Sheldon, 2000; Sherman, 2006; Smith, 2006; Zerwekh, 2006.

Several spiritual-religious topics deserve additional discussion concerning the nursing role in responding to patients' spiritual needs. These topics are prayer, forgiveness, relief from suffering, and various faith traditions.

Prayer

For patients at the end of life, coming to peace with God and prayer are often valued as much as good pain control (Steinhauser et al., 2000). Prayer is communication with God or the divine; 90% of Americans pray (Paloma & Gallup, 1991). Prayer can bring comfort, be a coping strategy, and lead to transcendence. You can ask patients what helps them to pray. Patients also may find it helpful when a nurse says, "I am praying for you" (Taylor & Outlaw, 2002). As an intervention, prayer is not "one size fits all," meaning the nurse needs to consider the uniqueness of the patient when facilitating prayer. One concern is the possibility of spiritual pain stemming from unanswered prayer (Taylor & Outlaw). Prayer should be consistent with a patient's beliefs and practices; introducing new or unfamiliar spiritual or religious practices may contribute to distress (Sherman, 2006). Because prayer is often considered personal and private, health care professionals may be hesitant to facilitate or introduce prayer—fearing rejection or a sense of spiritual inadequacy (Kemp, 2006). In these situations, patients can be referred to a chaplain, spiritual counselor, or a health professional who has developed expertise in spiritual care. Nurses may also offer a blessing that is not from a specific faith tradition.

Facilitating Forgiveness

Forgiving and being forgiven lead to inner peace, peace with others, and peace with God (Puchalski et al., 2004). Forgiveness is a voluntary letting go of anger, bitterness, resentment, and the need to retaliate after an injury; forgiveness leads to reconciliation (Mickley & Cowles, 2001; Festa & Tuck, 2000). Regret and guilt may be experienced as dying persons consider their relationships (Kemp, 2006). Forgiveness is one strategy for the healing of troubled relationships and can lead to closure at the end of life. Patients may be at various stages or phases in the process of forgiveness, which has implications for nursing interventions. Forgiveness involves examining the injury event, understanding it, reframing it, and letting it go. Mickley and Cowles analyzed the experience of forgiveness of 25 persons who were receiving palliative or terminal care; they identified four phases of forgiveness based on their data:

1. "I won't forgive"—endurance of the hurt with strong negative emotions.

2. "I can't forgive"—increase in tension between the negative emotions and personal values.

3. "Should I forgive?"—analysis of the situation.

4. "I have forgiven"—letting go of negative emotion and following personal values.

Offering yourself as a nonjudgmental listener can facilitate developing an awareness of the need for forgiveness in a relationship (Mickley & Cowles, 2001). Patients' definitions of forgiveness, values, and ideas of how to accomplish forgiveness are important considerations in how to support them in forgiveness work. Patients may also choose not to forgive (Mickley & Cowles).

Questions for Facilitating Forgiveness

- With whom would you like to be closer?
- What stands in the way and keeps you apart?
- If the relationship could be the way you wanted it to be, how would it be?
- What do you think might make it better?

Source: Festa & Tuck, 2000, p. 83

Responding to spiritual suffering

Coaching is an effective way to respond to the spiritual suffering of dying patients and their family members. "Coaching is an interpersonal intervention that requires the therapeutic use of the self, involving the mind, past experience, words, heart, and hands—to comfort those who suffer" (Spross, 1996, p. 201). As a coach, a nurse can relieve suffering by journeying with patients as a companion who recognizes the pain of their losses, reassures them that they will not be abandoned in their suffering, and facilitates expression of feelings to help them find meaning in suffering (Sherman, 2006).

Communication for Different Faith Traditions

Discussion of spiritual perspectives in this chapter is influenced by a Judeo-Christian perspective of beliefs and values, which underlies the philosophical traditions of health care in the United States. Assessing spiritual needs should help nurses tailor spiritual interventions to be consistent with the spiritual and religious practices of patients and families. Although a thorough analysis of different faith traditions is beyond the scope of this chapter, Table 4.1 shows some of the various perspectives we may encounter in providing spiritual care to patients. Keep in mind that variability also exists within each of the faith traditions. A nurse can show respect by asking patients and families to explain what spiritual practices are important to them.

Table 4.1   Religious Communication Considerations for Patients/ Families.

Buddhism

- Suffering can be eliminated by thinking right thoughts and avoiding self-centeredness.

- Death is not a moment; it is viewed as a transition and part of the cycle of life. Allow a 10-minute period of respect (not moving or talking around the body) following death.

- Talking about death is viewed as making death happen faster (instead of talking directly about death to the dying person or spouse, it might be better to talk with children or other relatives).

- Buddhists have a desire to remain conscious in order to think right thoughts.

Christianity

- Christians believe in eternal life; death is a positive transition to a better world.

- Christians generally welcome clergy, scripture reading, prayer, and hymns.

Hinduism

- God is internal and external, within every person and transcending every person.

- Hindus believe in the concept of reincarnation and view death as union with God.

- Hindus believe the life lived in this world influences the next life.

- Hindus experience comfort in positive life review.

Islam

- Prayer is practiced five times a day.

- Death represents a transition to eternal life with Allah; afterlife is preceded by the "Day of Decision" or "Day of Reckoning," at which time afterlife in paradise or hell will be determined.

continues

Table 4.1   Religious Communication Considerations for Patients/
Families.   *(continued)*

Islam

- Muslims view death as a temporary loss; excessive grieving may be viewed as inappropriate.
- Muslims may fear the dying process and may not welcome discussion about death.
- When death is near, the Qur'an is read at the bedside.

Judaism

- Life is highly valued as a gift from God; continuing to live a productive life is supported.
- Suffering can be punishing, teaching, or redemptive; may be concerned with the "why" of suffering.
- Emphasis is on the here and now rather than life beyond; beliefs about afterlife are varied, with some believing in no afterlife.

Sources: O'Brien, 2003; Sherman, 2006; Smith, 2001

The Spiritual Journey of Health Care Professionals

The spirituality of health care professionals certainly influences how they provide spiritual care. Sinclair, Raffin, Pereira, and Guebert (2006) explored the spirituality of 20 members of a palliative interdisciplinary team, half of whom were nurses. Palliative care provided an impetus for their own spiritual journeys for some participants. They viewed their work as a calling that provided fulfillment in their lives. They identified several challenges to experiencing spirituality in the workplace, including compassion fatigue, tension with role overlaps, and no clear assignment regarding spiritual care. Shared community values in caring for the dying contributed to a sense of belonging and a collective spirituality. Cornette

(2005) found that nurses, physicians, pastors, and volunteers who provided palliative care became more aware of their own spiritual lives. Caring for dying patients created a desire to enjoy the fullness of life.

Developing Competence in Spiritual Care

Participating in continuing interdisciplinary education on spiritual care is one strategy for increasing your ability to effectively provide spiritual care. Longaker, an educational director with a spiritual care program in London, developed a program titled "Wisdom and Compassion in Care for the Dying" for professionals and volunteers after recognizing and responding to the suffering of dying persons and their relatives. The program includes reflection on fears of death, techniques for active and compassionate listening, recognition of and response to emotional and spiritual suffering, and nondenominational spiritual practices such as contemplation and meditation (Wasner, Longaker, Fegg, & Borasio, 2005). Participation in the 3 ½ day program resulted in improved attitudes toward participants' families and colleagues, increased work satisfaction, and improved work atmosphere. Additional strategies for developing competence in spiritual care are

- Complete a spiritual assessment, using a structured assessment guideline.

- Role play a discussion about spiritual beliefs and values with attention to being respectful and nonjudgmental.

- Review and critique research about spirituality in health care.

- Review cases in which patients' spiritual beliefs affect health—discuss possible spiritual care interventions.

- Discuss roles of interdisciplinary health team members, including clergy.

- Reflect on own spiritual values.

- Participate in experiential learning activities: Create a self-epitaph, imagine being diagnosed with a terminal disease, identify needs and losses, and reflect on losses in your own life.

- Analyze how religious traditions affect end-of-life care (Beckman et al., 2007; Puchalski & Larson, 1998).

Providing spiritual care at the end of life, as with all aspects of end-of-life care, can be enhanced by collaborative interdisciplinary planning and interventions. Because nurses have a significant amount of face-to-face time as they provide care every day, they have frequent opportunities to integrate spiritual interventions into caring activities.

Reflective Practice

Spirituality and religion are perceived as private. Although worship often occurs with others and a supportive religious community affirms and validates spiritual and religious beliefs and values, people may fear that expressing faith and spiritual needs may be intrusive to others when in settings outside a religious community. When people are dying, they are certainly physically vulnerable and also may be vulnerable spiritually. Nurses deal with vulnerable bodies every day, and so it makes sense to both patients and nurses that nurses by necessity enter into that private space of bodies. Nurses' entering into the private space of spirituality in situations of vulnerability is less understood by the public as well as nurses. The fear of intrusion and lack of clarity about acceptable actions in spiritual care make us less certain about what actions we should take in responding to spiritual vulnerability.

"By having the courage to examine our own spirituality, we can develop the compassion needed to listen and be with dying persons on their own spiritual journey."

As we have emphasized, nurses who are uncomfortable with their spirituality will be less able to perceive and respond to the spiritual needs of their dying patients and family members. Given the nature of palliative care, which is focused on being with patients on their journey to the end of life, responding to spiritual needs and concerns is an essential component of care. For the nurse who feels called to palliative care, there is an obligation to develop competence in providing spiritual care. Whether or not we are comfortable with our own spiritual values, we should each examine how our spiritual beliefs and values influence our life choices and our nursing care of dying patients. This kind of reflection can help us understand the universal need for finding meaning and purpose in life and the search for spiritual and religious connections. By having the courage to examine our own spirituality, we can develop the compassion needed to listen and be with dying persons on their own spiritual journey.

Discomfort with religious beliefs and practices different from our own is likely, because we are often uncomfortable with what we don't understand or have not experienced. Gaining additional knowledge about religious beliefs and practices can diminish this discomfort and help us to be compassionate for others as we identify and respond to their spiritual needs at the end of life. This same discomfort can also interfere with our ability to dialogue with our colleagues about spiritual care. We may fear rejection or a lack of understanding from health care team members about spiritual care interventions. The easier thing to do is request a referral to a clergyperson, chaplain, or other spiritual counselor. That is important, but we must keep in mind that spiritual care can be provided every day in many of the encounters we have with dying persons. All members of palliative care teams need to work collectively to identify and offer spiritual care strategies that respond to the unique spiritual needs and concerns of their dying patients.

Ethical Practice in Facilitating Forgiveness

ETHICAL PROBLEM: What should I do when my dying patient is estranged from her daughter because of past family conflicts?

What should I value?

- Respecting the patient's privacy.

- A good death for the patient.

- A sense of closure or peace in the relationship for the patient and her daughter.

Who should I be?

- A compassionate listener.

- A compassionate nurse who identifies and responds to the patient's spiritual needs.

What should I do?

- Ask nonthreatening questions that help the patient reflect on what she wants in the relationship with her daughter such as, "What stands in the way and keeps you apart?" or "What do you think might make this better?"

- Reflect to the patient your observations of the distress the patient is showing about the troubled relationship.

- Explore strategies with the patient that could facilitate forgiveness and reconciliation in the relationship.

- Ask the patient if it would be helpful to talk to a chaplain or other spiritual counselor.

- Support patient's choices that will contribute to a peaceful death.

Nurses' Stories

Spiritual Pain, Distress, and Suffering

Our focus in caring for dying patients is on providing symptom relief and comfort. Sometimes common interventions such as opioids for pain and other medications for anxiety do not address the true cause of the distress. A hospice nurse relates an experience with a patient who was not responding to pain intervention.

> We kept upping her dose of morphine, but it didn't seem to touch her pain. Finally our hospice chaplain said, "Maybe something else is going on." So the next time I saw her, I asked if she was afraid of something. It took some time, but she finally told me that she had been raised Roman Catholic but had divorced an abusive husband. She thought she'd been expelled from the church because of her divorce and now was afraid to die and have to be buried in unconsecrated ground. Well, I asked the hospice chaplain to help me, and he arranged for a priest to come and welcome her back into the church. Miraculously, her pain went away. If the chaplain hadn't worked with me, I don't think I would have ever gotten her pain under control.

Healing While Dying

Patients who are dying say they want to be recognized as a whole being with the ability to contribute. Contribution sometimes means reconciliation, forgiving, and being forgiven. A hospice nurse tells of working with an elderly patient who was often abrupt and rude.

> We were trying out this new assessment form called a suffering assessment. I didn't want to ask him the questions because I thought he'd be gruff and tell me this was "stupid," so I gave him the form and said he could fill it out if he felt like it. He read it and when he came to the question "How much are you suffering due to personal and family issues," he marked down a 10 (the most suffering possible). When I asked him about it, he told me he had lost touch with his son and wanted to see him again. I think he needed his son's forgiveness.

"Spirituality can be defined as the quest for meaning, while religion is a structured belief system that is a component of spirituality."

Spiritual Competency

Competency in spiritual care can be developed just as other technical skills can be mastered. Competency includes recognizing that each patient has individual spiritual and religious needs. An ICU nurse commented on spirituality:

> I think spirituality is a delicate matter. I've gotten to respect it more over the years. [Although] I'm not ... comfortable offering to pray with patients, I feel we have to respect all sides of a person. In their dying time, their spirituality is so important. I have to be very cautious, because I sometimes think people think they have to pray. [But they can be the one who decides.] It's their agenda.

Key Points

- Spirituality can be defined as the quest for meaning, while religion is a structured belief system that is a component of spirituality.

- Spiritual needs of dying patients can include maintaining a sense of self-worth, leaving a legacy, forgiveness, and reconciliation.

- Spiritual distress can manifest itself in physical distress such as pain, anxiety, and other symptoms.

- Nurses have a significant role to play in addressing spiritual needs of dying patients and can develop competence in this area.

REFLECTION QUESTIONS

1. How does your own sense of spirituality and religious practices influence how you care for patients at the end of life?

2. What does it mean to have healing while dying?

3. Think about a specific patient who is approaching the end of life. What questions and strategies can you use to have a conversation about the patient's spiritual needs?

References

Anandarajah, G., & Hight, E. (2001). Spirituality and medical practice: Using the HOPE questions as a practical tool for spiritual assessment. *American Family Physician, 63*(1), 81-88.

Beckman, S., Baxley-Harges, S., Bruick-Sorge, C., & Salmon, B. (2007). Five strategies that heighten nurses' awareness of spirituality to impact client care. *Holistic Nursing Practice, 21*(3), 135-139.

Cassell, E. J. (1991). *The nature of suffering and the goals of medicine.* New York: Oxford University Press.

Cavendish, R., Edelman, M., Naradovy, L., Bajo, M. M., Perosi, I., & Lanza, M. (2007). Do pastoral care providers recognize nurses as spiritual care providers? *Holistic Nursing Practice, 21*(2), 89-98.

Chochinov, H. M., & Cann, B. J. (2005). Interventions to enhance the spiritual aspects of dying. *Journal of Palliative Medicine, 8*(Suppl. 1), S103-S115.

Cornette, K. (2005). For whenever I am weak, I am strong. *International Journal of Palliative Nursing, 11*(3), 147-153.

Doka, K. (1993). The spiritual needs of the dying. In K. Doka & J. Morgan (Eds.), *Death and spirituality* (pp. 143-150). Amityville, NY: Baywood.

Festa, L. M., & Tuck, I. (2000). A review of forgiveness literature with implications for nursing practice. *Holistic Nursing Practice, 14*(4), 77-86.

Gauthier, D. M. (2002). The meaning of healing near the end of life. *Journal of Hospice and Palliative Nursing, 4*(4), 220-227.

Grant, D. (2004). Spiritual interventions: How, when, and why nurses use them. *Holistic Nursing Practice, 18*, 36-41.

Hermann, C. P. (2006). Development and testing of the spiritual needs inventory for patients near the end of life. *Oncology Nursing Forum, 33*(4), 737-744.

Hermann, C. P. (2007). The degree to which spiritual needs of patients near the end of life are met. *Oncology Nursing Forum, 34*(1), 70-78.

Highfield, M. (2000). Providing spiritual care to patients with cancer. *Clinical Journal of Oncology Nursing, 4*(3), 115-120.

Holmes, S. M., Rabow, M. W., & Dibble, S. L. (2006). Screening the soul: Communication regarding spiritual concerns among primary care physicians and seriously ill patients approaching the end of life. *American Journal of Hospice and Palliative Medicine, 23*(1), 25-33.

Hudson, R., & Rumbold, B. (2003). Spiritual care. In M. O'Connor & S. Aranda, (Eds.) *Palliative care nursing: A guide to practice* (pp. 69-86). Melbourne, Australia: Ausmed Publications.

Kemp, C. (2006). Spiritual care interventions. In B. R. Ferrell & N. Coyle, (Eds.). *Textbook of palliative care nursing* (pp. 595-604). New York: Oxford University Press.

Lunn, J. S. (2003). Spiritual care in a multi-religious context. *Journal of Pain & Palliative Care Pharmacotherapy, 17*, 153-166.

McEwan, M. (2005). Spiritual nursing care: State of the art. *Holistic Nursing Practice, 19*, 161-168.

Mickley, J. R., & Cowles, K. (2001). Ameliorating the tension: Use of forgiveness and healing. *Oncology Nursing Forum, 28*(1), 31-37.

Murata, H. (2003). Spiritual pain and its care in patients with terminal cancer: Construction and conceptual framework by philosophical approach. *Palliative and Supportive Care, 1*, 15-21.

Murray, S. A. (2004). Exploring the spiritual needs of people dying of lung cancer or heart failure: A prospective quality interview study of patients and their carers. *Palliative Medicine, 18,* 39-45.

O'Brien, M. E. (2003). *Spirituality in nursing: Standing on holy ground.* Sudbury, MA: Jones and Bartlett.

O'Connor, P. (1993). A clinical paradigm for exploring spiritual concerns. In K. Doka & J. Morgan (Eds.), *Death and spirituality* (pp. 133-150). Amityville, NY: Baywood.

O'Gorman, M. L. (2002). Spiritual care at the end of life. *Critical Care Nursing Clinics of North America, 14,* 171-176.

Paloma, M. M., & Gallup, G. H. Jr. (1991). *Varities of prayer: A survey report.* Philadelphia: Trinity Press International.

Puchalski, C. (1999). Spiritual assessment tool (FICA). *Spirituality and end-of-life care, 1*(6). Retrieved June 27, 2008, from http://www2.edc.org/lastacts/assess.asp

Puchalski, C., & Larson, D. (1998). Developing curricula in spirituality and medicine. *Academic Medicine, 73,* 970-974.

Puchalski, C. M., Dorff, E., & Hendi, Y. (2004). Spirituality, religion, and healing in palliative care. *Clinics in Geriatric Medicine, 20,* 689-714.

Robinson, M. R., Thiel, M. M., Backus, M. M., & Meyer, E. C. (2006). Matters of spirituality at the end of life in the pediatric intensive care unit. *Pediatrics, 118*(3), e719-e729.

Ryan, S. (1997). Chaplains are more than what chaplains do. *Visions, 3*(7), 8-9.

Sessanna, L., Finnell, D., & Jezewski, M. A. (2007). Spirituality in nursing and health-related literature. *Journal of Holistic Nursing, 25*(4), 252-262.

Sexson, S. B. (2004). Religious and spiritual assessment of the child and adolescent. *Child and Adolescent Psychiatric Clinics of North America, 13,* 35-47.

Sheldon, J. E. (2000). Spirituality as a part of nursing. *Journal of Hospice and Palliative Nursing, 2*(3), 101-108.

Shelly, J. A. (2000). *Spiritual care: A guide for caregivers.* Downers Grove, IL: Intervarsity Press.

Sherman, D. W. (2006). Spirituality and culture as domains of quality palliative care. In M. L. Matzo & D. W. Sherman (Eds.), *Palliative care nursing: Quality care to the end of life* (pp. 3-49). New York: Springer Publishing.

Sinclair, S., Raffin, S., Pereira, J., & Guebert, N. (2006). Collective soul: The spirituality of an interdisciplinary palliative care team. *Palliative and Supportive Care, 4,* 13-24.

Smith, A. R. (2006). Using the Synergy Model to provide spiritual nursing care in critical care settings. *Critical Care Nurse, 26*(4), 41-47.

Smith, D. (2001). Spiritual perspectives in end of life care. In B. Poor & G. P. Poirrier, (Eds.). *End of life nursing care* (pp. 201-209). Sudbury, MA: Jones and Bartlett.

Spross, J. (1996). Coaching and suffering: The role of the nurse in helping people face illness. In B. R. Ferrell (Ed.), *Suffering* (pp. 159-171). Sudbury, MA: Jones and Bartlett.

Steinhauser, K. E., Clipp, E. C., McNeilly, M., Christakis, N., McIntryre, L. M., & Tulsky, J. A. (2000). In search of a good death: Observations of patients, families, and providers. *Annals of Internal Medicine, 12*(10), 825-832.

Stoll, R. I. (1979). Guidelines for spiritual assessment. *American Journal of Nursing, 79,* 1574-1577.

Taylor, E. J. (2006). Spiritual assessment. In B. R. Ferrell & N. Coyle (Eds.). *Textbook of palliative care nursing* (pp. 581-594). New York: Oxford University Press.

Taylor, E. J., & Outlaw, F. H. (2002). Use of prayer among persons with cancer. *Holistic Nursing Practice, 16*(3), 46-60.

Van der Poel, C. J. (1998). *Sharing the journey: Spiritual assessment and pastoral response to persons with incurable illnesses.* Collegeville, MN: Liturgical Press.

Wasner, M., Longaker, C., Fegg, M. J., & Borasio, G. D. (2005). Effects of spiritual care training for palliative care professionals. *Palliative Medicine, 19,* 99-104.

Williams, A. (2006). Perspectives on spirituality at the end of life: A meta-summary. *Palliative and Supportive Care, 4,* 407-417.

Zalenski, R. J., & Raspa, R. (2006). Maslow's hierarchy of needs: A framework for achieving human potential in hospice. *Journal of Palliative Medicine, 9*(5), pp. 1120-1127.

Zerwekh, J. V. (2006). *Nursing care at the end of life.* Philadelphia: F. A. Davis.

My first reaction is to take the patient advocacy role. I recall a situation with a patient. He had five kids, and he had a brain tumor. All the kids were in different places, emotionally. I walked into the home, and the patient was fine. He was happy, on a lot of steroids, was eating well, and he was comfortable. The five children were there, and one of them was the note taker—he wanted to make sure that every avenue had been explored. The patient wasn't able to express what he wanted, so I thought of myself as the advocate. The family was fighting, and it got very intense. What it came down to was that the doctor had said they could do more chemotherapy. Some of the kids wanted it, and others wanted him left alone. I called the doctor and talked with him and set it up so the family could come in and talk with him. They talked about what kind of chemo he could have. Two of the kids wanted to do the chemo and wanted to know how soon they could start. Then, I asked the doctor, "In your best experience, how effective would this chemo be?" I had prepped the doctor, and he was ready for the question. "I think it's a 0.5 or 1.3 percent chance." And the son said, "Is that all?" Then the family decided they didn't want it.

—Hospice Nurse

5

·

Responding to
Conflict

One of the most challenging aspects for nurses in caring for patients as they are dying is dealing with conflict. We are faced not only with our patients and their families at a time of high emotion and difficult decisions, but we also face our own values and beliefs and the values and beliefs of other health care team members. Often, we are not all in agreement about what is the best course for our patients.

Conflict and Its Consequences

Conflict is a part of life. It is inevitable in a world made up of unique individuals. For nurses, conflict may happen between a nurse and a patient or family, between a nurse and a physician, or between staff members on a health care team (Dahlin & Gianiracusa, 2006). For patients, conflict may occur with other family members or with health care staff. Conflict can be beneficial, because it can help people see different points of view and result in positive change. Conflict may become worse, it may be avoided, or the people involved may try to resolve it.

Potential Consequences of Unresolved Conflict in End-of-Life Care

- Fragmentation of care, leading to patient suffering.

- Exhaustion, emotional depletion, and stress.

- Poor communication.

- Delay in making decisions, which may contribute to inefficient use of resources, as well as increased suffering.

- Guilt and embarrassment because of unresolved conflict.

- Patient and family confusion, anxiety, and distress.

- Moral distress for health care professionals when they are expected to provide care that conflicts with values.

- Not considering the perspectives of others.

- Interpreting the responses of others based on your own hurt, anger, or fear.

- Frustration, tension, burnout, or job dissatisfaction for health care staff.

- For professionals, leaving the job.

- Escalation of conflict.

Sources: Elpern, Covert, & Kleinpell, 2005; Pattison, 2004; Bowman, 2000b; Mari, Farrell, Lacroix, Graeme, & Shemie, 2000.

When two people or groups perceive they are in conflict, a possible response is to move further to the opposite side of the conflict issue. An "I am right and you are wrong" attitude can result. Each side might overstate or exaggerate its case in an effort to make a strong point. Overstating your case or avoiding the conflict may lead to a failure to see the perspectives of others involved in the conflict and is likely to increase the distance between the people involved (Bowman, 2000b).

In a study of intensive care unit (ICU) patients who were to have treatment withheld or withdrawn, 78% experienced conflict (Breen, Abernethy, Abbott, & Tulsky, 2001). Nearly half of the family members who participated in discussions about end-of-life decisions reported they experienced conflict, most frequently with ICU clinicians (Abbott, Sago, Breen, Abernethy, & Tulsky, 2001).

Sources of Conflict in End-of-Life Care

The challenge of making choices for health care at the end of life is in itself a potential conflict-generating situation. These decisions have consequences for life and death; lead to thinking about the meaning of life; and often involve values, morality, ethical principles, and legal issues. These areas can bring about intense emotions and increase the potential for conflict (Bowman, 2000a). A study on a model for resolving end-of-life care disputes found that the conflicts did not involve distrust of the health care system. Rather, conflicts were often focused on treatment goals and prognosis; most of the conflict occurred either within the treatment team or between the treatment team and members of the patient-family group (Buchanan, Desrochers, Henry, Thomassen, & Barrett, Jr., 2002). Conflicts resulted from different perceptions, interpretations, and values related to end-of-life decisions.

"Family member tensions can easily emerge when confronting the difficult decisions involved in end-of-life care."

Family members can be at different points in accepting the prognosis of their dying family member, resulting in a lack of consensus about treatment or non-treatment choices. An example is when family members interpret the reality of the situation differently. They may not be in agreement about how much information should be given to the dying patient, because some members may believe that the patient will lose hope and give up (Stanley & Zoloth-Dorfman, 2006).

Family member tensions can easily emerge when confronting the difficult decisions involved in end-of-life care. In a study on tensions uncovered in family conferences in the ICU setting, researchers found that contradictions occurred either between family members or among individual family members. Persons involved in end-of-life care decisions may experience internal conflict about possible choices and how to make decisions. The overarching tension identified in the study focused on whether or not the family should allow the patient to die naturally, in the present, or to extend the patient's life with artificial means (Hsieh, Shannon, & Curtis, 2006).

Two important sources of conflict directly related to communication include communication breakdowns among family and health care professionals and lack of information (Abbott et al., 2001; Boyle, Miller, & Forbes-Thompson, 2005; Buchanan et al., 2002). Health care staff may fail to recognize what information is important to patients and families, or their daily work may not allow them adequate time to inquire about and meet the needs that patients and families have for information. At the same time, family members are likely experiencing high levels of stress related to the need to make care decisions, which can lead to physical and emotional exhaustion (Bowman, 2000b). Health care professionals are often more concerned about accuracy of clinical judgment and the benefit of treatment than understanding the beliefs and values of patients and families. While health care professionals may more often approach end-of-life decisions from a rational, cognitive approach, if they do not pay attention to the emotional component of end-of-life decisions, conflict can result.

The findings of a Dutch ethnographic study on communication between patients and clinic staff (The, Hak, Koeter, & van der Wal, 2000) indicate this cognitive-affective tension. Patients with lung cancer experienced conflict about wanting the truth about their prognosis versus not wanting to know. Although physicians explained to patients that the illness could not be cured, the physicians also offered treatment that, for patients, resulted in false optimism about cure. Physicians acted from a cognitive perspective, while the emotional status of the patients prevented them from acknowledging the reality of the terminal nature of the illness. Of great importance is for all involved in decision-making to pay adequate attention to both the cognitive perspective in understanding the reality of the information, and the emotional perspective in acknowledging how patients feel about what is happening to them.

Different perspectives about end-of-life care decisions are developed by patients and families in comparison to predominant perspectives more typical of health care professionals, who experience the environment of the health care system on a daily basis. Varying perspectives result from difference in age, social class, culture, and education (Bowman, 2000a). In addition, health professionals may experience time constraints for making decisions and acting on those decisions that can interfere with a timely decision-making process. What is valued by health care staff may be outside the understanding of patients and families or not important to them. These conflicting perspectives may become evident when a major decision for care needs becomes imperative. Health care teams may actually perceive that family members are difficult and impede the process of good decision-making, while family members are likely to have little understanding of the complexity and culture of ICUs or the health care system (Bowman, 2000a; Dawson, 2008).

Conflict Among Health Care Team Members

Members of the health care team also have experienced different educational approaches that can lead to conflict among the various disciplines and their related roles in caring for the dying. Physicians may be biased toward keeping death at a distance, and they may perceive death as a professional failure (Asch-Goodkin, 2000). In addition, if a patient's prognosis is difficult to predict, conflict may result about what to do (Dawson, 2008). Physicians often focus on prognosis, while nurses tend to focus on quality of life. For nurses, conflict often occurs when they must provide the care the physician orders, but they perceive the care to be futile and inflicting unnecessary pain on the patient (Badger, 2005). Frequent changes in team members and in care-delivery systems can lead to different understandings and fragmented communication between health care team members, increasing the likelihood of conflict (Bowman, 2000a).

Sources of Conflict in End-of-Life Care

Family

- Existing family dysfunction.
- Changing roles in family dynamics.
- Not knowing what to expect.
- Family members are at different levels of acceptance of prognosis.
- Extreme stress and fatigue.
- Lack of information about prognosis.
- Family members have different values about what is important at the end of life in comparison to one another and in comparison to health care professionals.

Health Care Professionals

- Different approaches to education of health professionals influence their values and approaches to end-of-life care.
- Time constraints for deciding, acting, and determining outcomes.
- Disease or illness presents a difficult prognosis.
- Differing opinions about care or treatment perspectives among health care providers compete against a patient's expressed wishes.
- Patient and family member perspectives are overlooked.
- Health care team members have negative views about the contribution of family members to treatment or care decision-making.
- Communication between the patient and family members is fragmented.

Health Care System

- Complexity and culture may not be understood by the patient and family.
- A fast-paced and high-performance ("success" oriented) environment makes it challenging to find the time to systematically address conflict.
- Organizational culture is nonsupportive of conflict resolution.
- System may be revenue-focused and biased toward continuing treatment and care as long as possible.

Ethical Conflict

We experience ethical conflict when we are troubled about doing the right thing (Cameron, 1993). Researchers have specifically explored the ethical problems experienced by health care professionals who provide end-of-life care. In a qualitative study of Canadian physicians and nurses, Oberle (2001) found that the core ethical problem for members of both professions was witnessing suffering, along with a sense of obligation to relieve or reduce suffering. Uncertainty about the best course of action led to moral distress about what to do. Because of the different professional roles, physicians viewed themselves as responsible for decisions, while nurses indicated they had to live with those decisions. All of the nurses (n=14) reported they experienced moral distress from conflict with physicians and the inability to influence care decisions, while none of the physicians reported moral distress from conflicts with nurses. For physicians, ethical conflict resulted from the hierarchical organizational structure of hospitals, which they perceived as interfering with their ability to make the best decisions for patients.

Jezuit (2000) explored the suffering of six critical care nurses who worked in a U.S. medical center. The nurses experienced conflict with physicians, family members, and within themselves. They had ethical conflict about comforting rather than "killing" the patient, as well as knowing when to intervene in family conflict. The nurses also found that support from medical staff was lacking and felt helpless and angry about patients' suffering. The struggle to balance their personal and professional responsibilities with obligations to patients generated conflict that added to nurse suffering (Rushton, 1992; Stanley & Zoloth-Dorfman, 2006). In another U.S. study of 28 medical intensive care unit nurses, responses to a moral distress scale (MDS) indicated the highest level of distress came from nurses required to provide aggressive care to patients they perceived as not benefiting from such care (Elpern, Covert, & Kleinpell, 2005). Zuzelo (2007) used the same MDS with a sample of 100 U.S. nurses (60% in critical care) and found that nurses experienced distress when family wishes to continue life support were followed even though the life support did not serve the patient's best interests. In an analysis of short answer questions in Zuzelo's study, five of eight themes were associated with end-of-life care situations:

1. resentment of physicians' reluctance to address death and dying,

2. going against or ignoring patients' wishes (about unwanted treatment),

3. worrying that quality of life issues were ignored during decision-making,

4. feeling frustrated with family members (for overriding requests of patients or refusing to end aggressive care when it was not helpful), and

5. seeing patients treated as experiments.

The differing perspectives of physicians and nurses also contributed to the ethical issues experienced by nurses who cared for terminally ill elderly adults in England (Enes & de Vries, 2004). Nurses reported situations in which they did not agree with physicians' decisions about artificial feeding, transferring patients to the hospital for active treatment, or using antibiotics. The researchers suggested that conflict between doctors and nurses results from professional hierarchy and power differentials, as well as different professional roles. Given these differences, nurses may believe their role in decision-making about treatment plans is minimal, and they may not question the medical plan of care (Enes & de Vries). In an analysis of differences in physician and nurse perspectives on end-of life decisions, Ferrand and colleagues (2003) found nurses did not feel included in decision-making, and they believed that a lack of cohesion or agreement actually delayed discussion about the need to stop or not begin treatment to sustain life.

In the study by Enes and de Vries (2004), only 3 out of 135 nurses identified conflicts between patients and families about giving information and accepting that the patient was dying, while Schaffer (2007) found that interactions with family members were the most frequently identified ethical conflict for Norwegian health professionals who provided end-of-life care (27% of all ethical problems identified). The analysis of interviews (17 of 25 were nurses) resulted in eight categories of ethical problems, indicating situations of ethical conflict:

1. interacting with family members,

2. quality of health care services,

3. disagreement among health care professionals,

4. treatment decisions,

5. involving elders in decision-making,

6. reluctance to talk about death,

7. managing own feelings and burdens of caregiving, and

8. meeting spiritual needs.

Autonomy Versus Beneficence

Autonomy for the patient alone is not adequate for ethical decision-making. If patient autonomy is the only consideration in end-of-life decisions, conflict will happen. An individual exists in relationship to an entire community, which in the case of end-of-life care includes family members and health care staff (Ladd, Pasquella, & Smith, 2000). Because of education and culture, most nurses and physicians in the United States view patient autonomy as primary in decision-making about end-of-life care (Bowman, 2000a). However, it is relevant to consider everyone's perspective, which is respecting the autonomy of each person involved.

Robertson (1996) found that physicians and nurses have different views about the importance of autonomy. Nurses were more likely to emphasize patient autonomy, while physicians emphasized beneficence—the good that would be achieved from treatment. However, dismissing or not giving importance to a patient's preferences, because of concern for what the best treatment is for a patient, is a response that may be more about medical paternalism than about empowering patients to make informed decisions (Breier-Mackie, 2001). Nurses desired to support patient autonomy by helping them to live in normal and independent ways during their care. However, supporting a patient's autonomy may not always result in the most good for a patient if that patient is not realistic about the situation.

To balance autonomy and beneficence, or to resolve the tension or conflict between these two ethical principles, nurses should reflect both on what a patient wants and what actions will promote good outcomes for that patient. Finding this balance involves inquiry and reflection about what a patient and family desire and why, as well as how health care provider perspectives contribute to the process of decision-making. In doing so, the role of the nurse becomes one of patient advocacy (see Chapter 6); finding balance also may mean a nurse needs to seek a "middle ground" that takes into account patient, family, and physician perspectives (Breier-Mackie, 2001).

Futility

Care is considered futile if it is not consistent with goals of patients, medical practice, or community standards for care (Miller, Funk, & Wiegand, 2006). In some situations, the care is futile from the clinician's perspective only, which means that specific treatment is perceived as valuable by a patient or family but is not clinically indicated. In other situations, the care may be clinically indicated, but the patient or family does not see value in proceeding with treatment (Breier-Mackie, 2001; Pattison, 2004). However, futility is often a judgment call and as such can generate conflict about the right thing to do. In some situations, determining when additional interventions will not result in any improvement and at what point a person is dying is challenging (Weaver, 2004). Care is never futile, but medical interventions sometimes are.

Responding to Conflict

Hsieh et al. (2006) categorized communication strategies for responding to tensions in family conferences about end-of-life decisions for intensive-care patients as information-seeking and decision-centered strategies. The contradictions experienced by people involved in end-of-life decision-making may be resolved through providing current and accurate information, which can prevent a conflict situation from developing. *Information-seeking strategies* include the following actions:

- acknowledging,
- clarifying,
- re-centering (to another focus),
- reaffirming (gives value to both sides),
- recalibrating (moves from an oppositional framework), and
- segmenting (dividing information into smaller compartments).

Decision-Centered Strategies

Decision-centered strategies involve supporting or not supporting a position and in some cases, the avoidance of making a decision. Information-seeking strategies work best when patients and family members are still trying to understand the contradictions or tensions involved in possible choices, while decision-centered strategies can support families in the decision-making process once they have resolved or reflected on the contradictions of the situation. It is important to involve multiple family members in the decision-making process, unless inconsistent with cultural practices, to gain emotional and practical support during a challenging process. Family members also need to be encouraged not to feel guilty for outcomes that result from the decision-making (Hsieh et al., 2006).

Consideration of family stressors can reduce conflict through understanding the experience of family members. By applying the family stress framework, the nurse can inquire about how family members understand the illness of the patient (perceptions); encourage the family to connect with helpful friends, other family members, and religious resources; and assess ways to strengthen family-member coping strategies.

Conflict Resolution Strategies

Preventing the development of conflict in the first place is ideal. (See sidebar, "Strategies for Reducing the Incidence of Conflict." Once a conflict has developed, the first step in resolution is to work toward understanding patient and family perspectives about their experience—beliefs about the cause, treatment, and outcomes. The next step is negotiating a treatment plan acceptable to all, which will be enhanced by open and clear communication (Bowman, 2000a). Kendall and Arnold (#184, n.d.) outline four steps of negotiation specific to end-of-life decision-making:

1. Separate people from the problem.

2. Focus on interests (everyone usually wants what is best for the patient).

3. Invent solutions (balance meeting family expectations and providing good medical care).

4. Outline objective criteria (for established goals).

Strategies for Reducing the Incidence of Conflict

- Provide current and accurate information about prognosis, treatment options, and expected outcomes.
- Respect cultural differences.
- Address own emotional responses.
- Develop self-awareness and inventory own biases and perspectives.
- Remember that persons involved in decision-making may be at different stages of acceptance of the situation.
- Identify the main spokesperson for the patient and family.
- Dialogue with other health care team members about the ethical aspects of decision-making.
- Strive for openness and transparency in communication.
- Reflect on how interactions with self and health care system may contribute to conflict.
- Clarify potential consequences of treatment and nontreatment options.
- Explore and identify interests and preferences of all involved.
- Pay attention to nonverbal cues of response to discussion of decisions.
- Work to understand patients or families' stories and contributions of emotional responses to decision-making.
- Encourage all involved to acknowledge feelings.

Conflict With Parents of Dying Children

- Be compassionate and avoid rushing parents into a decision.
- Explain that everyone is concerned about the child's best interests.
- Identify one person as the spokesperson to communicate about health care status and treatment options.
- Meet with parents frequently.
- Listen carefully to what is presented to the parents—work to understand their perceptions and values.
- Explain choices and the benefits and burdens associated with each choice.
- As possible, provide accurate data on prognosis.
- Explain that stopping or not beginning life-sustaining measures does not mean that the well-being of the child is being abandoned.

Sources: Dahlin & Gianiracusa, 2006; Hsieh et al., 2006; Bolmsjo & Heremeren, 2003; Burt, 2002; Oberle, 2001; Mari et al., 2000; Bowman, 2000b; Kendall & Arnold, #183, n.d.

Mediation

If conflict has developed that cannot be resolved through information-seeking and negotiation strategies, mediation may be needed. Mediation is a formal process with a neutral facilitator who can guide the discussion and decision-making. In a pilot project that showed the effectiveness of early, informal mediation in preventing future conflict, most of the conflict in the 12 cases involved intrafamily disagreement rather than disagreements between families and treatment teams (Buchanan et al., 2002). Bowman (2000b) suggests implementing pre-mediation steps that include:

- Normalize the conflict (acknowledge that conflict happens to everyone, and the difficult task of giving care at the end of life may contribute to conflict).

- Acknowledge the voluntary nature of settlement (not having to settle but wanting to settle should be acknowledged by those involved in the conflict).

- Consider differences between power and hierarchy (family and health care system).

- Assess whether cultural differences are part of the conflict (may need to use a cross-cultural approach to mediation).

Use of the pre-mediation model can increase the likelihood of success for a more formal mediation process, which involves the following steps (Bowman, 2000b):

- Negotiate ground rules.

- Identify the costs of the conflict (e.g., time, money, relationships, lack of progress in decision-making).

- Appeal to a higher responsibility (recognize effects of conflict on others).

- Clarify what is really being said (listen carefully).

- Identify the meaning of the conflict.

- Look for the affect (emotions).

- Act as a messenger (repeat what is being said).

- Find a shared purpose.

- Test the choices for outcome (beyond winning or losing).

- Develop solutions that show the larger picture (promoting change for better systems).

When conflict situations are particularly complex and intense, consultants, a professional advocate, or an ethics committee can help to determine a prudent course of action to resolve or reduce the conflict (American Medical Association, 1999).

Models of Care

Implementing models of care that establish a palliative care framework, as opposed to a critical care framework that is focused only on cure, can also reduce the development of conflict related to end-of-life care. Rushton, Williams, and Sabatier (2002) contrast the disintegration that is characteristic of the critical care environment with the integration of the palliative care approach. In a disintegrated environment, a person is sometimes "broken down" into component parts—the focus is on organs, data, and technology rather than on the whole person. An integrated environment that is focused on integrity of the person and system involves the following characteristics:

- Meaningful communication that promotes learning about patient values and preferences.

- View of the patient as a whole person, rather than independent, isolated systems.

- Presence of ethical reflection and ethical decision-making strategies.

- Respect for both medical and nursing models of care as well as what each health professional brings to the environment.

- Healing (spiritual and psychosocial) as the goal, rather than curing or eradicating disease.

"Sometimes we have the strength to support others, and sometimes we are the ones who need support."

Pattison (2004) also describes a model for integrating critical care and palliative care at the end of life. Reduction of the person, a "medicalized" approach to end-of life care, and fragmentation of care are predominant in critical care environments. Nurses have the capabilities to implement a holistic practice and function as "catalysts" to move the focus to palliative care that is comfort-oriented and patient- and family-centered. Pattison suggests that collaboration and advocacy (see Chapter 6) are nursing actions that not only resolve conflict but also can move the health care system toward providing better end-of-life care.

Reflective Practice

Conflict can sometimes surprise us, because we may be unaware of another's experience. We may think our care is good, and yet it might not be what another is experiencing—for people we work with or for people receiving our nursing care. Conflict can be scary, because sometimes we feel attacked—or feel we are inadequate. We may react with anger because we believe the reaction of another is unjust from our point of view. And if it is a conflict we have experienced before, our reaction may be "Oh, no—not again!" or "I don't think I can go through this again." Too often, we may react by avoiding people, or in extreme cases, by quitting a job because of the oppressive feeling conflict may bring.

Can we reframe that conflict to one of opportunity? Conflict brings opportunities to learn to understand others and initiate positive change. It can be an exercise in self-awareness—sometimes painful self-awareness. If we can take on the challenge, conflict can be a tremendous learning opportunity. We can gain an understanding of how our own views and actions may contribute to conflict. We can learn ways to identify signs of conflict and work toward early resolution before relationships are damaged by angry words or actions.

In end-of-life care, we know our patients and families are vulnerable. Daily interactions that normally might not cause conflict can result in an angry eruption.

Our own ability to manage conflict can vary from day to day. Sometimes we feel ready to take on challenges, and other times we don't. We need to be aware of our vulnerability as well as consider the vulnerability of our co-workers in managing conflict. Sometimes we have the strength to support others, and sometimes we are the ones who need support.

Ethical conflict can be especially challenging, because it often hits the very core of our being—our beliefs and values. It is only with understanding the beliefs and values of those on the other side of the conflict that we can make sense of why others would think differently about the right thing to do. Remember that good communication may resolve the conflict or at least result in an "agree to disagree" response. Nurses may not understand why doctors keep pushing for treatment. If we remember that age and education influence how doctors offer treatment, that response can be better understood. Understanding does not absolve us from responding to the conflict, but at least we can let others know we can understand why they might have a different viewpoint.

Nurses who are equipped with ethical language are better able to confront the conflict (using the virtue of courage) and explore what actions support both what the patient wants (autonomy) and what is best for the patient (beneficence). It takes time to do this, because we must give time to hear the stories of others to understand how they see the situation. However, that time can be well-spent for patients and families who are able to move more smoothly into care that is not futile or that contributes to additional suffering. By working toward the same goal, we will use resources more effectively and provide better patient care. In addition, the work environment is more likely to be positively energized by the synergy that results from colleagues sharing good work.

Nurses' Stories

Conflict With Physicians or Other Health Care Team Members

What do you do when you are not in agreement with a physician's treatment? Advocating for a patient can be difficult when you are not in agreement with the plan of care. Consider this hospice liaison nurse who wanted to assure that her hospitalized patient was not in pain:

> She had pain out of control, and when I got there they were trying to do an X-ray on her. I walked over to her bed and we looked at each other. I took her hand and she said to me, "Make these people leave." She was trying to tell me that she knew she was dying and her son was being released from prison to see her. All she wanted was to see him before she died. Her pain was increasing, and she needed more pain medication. The GI doctor came in, checked her bowels, and said, "There's nothing more we can do." I followed him out and asked him if we could increase her pain medication. He said, 'I'm not giving her that dose; it will kill her.'" Well, I wasn't about to let this go, so I followed him all the way down the hall. He looked at me and said, "What do you want now?" I said to him, "I'm sure you'd agree that this woman is not going to be with us much longer." I kept talking and talking. Finally I saw a little crack, so I said, "Sometimes when I'm in this situation I think, if this was my family member, what would I do?" He went back and wrote the order. The patient died peacefully the next day. I saw the doctor 2 weeks later, and he called me over and told me that his sister died a really horrible death years earlier, and he hadn't forgiven himself because he was the doctor and hadn't done anything. What's more, he was afraid of death. He needed somebody pressing him to make it okay.

In this situation, the nurse was gentle but persistent. She was able to resolve the conflict by keeping it framed in terms of what was best for the patient.

Ethical Practice in Responding to Conflict

ETHICAL PROBLEM: What should I do when the physician is pushing for aggressive treatment that a patient is reluctant to pursue?

What should I value?

- The patient's autonomy.
- The physician's autonomy.
- The physician's knowledge about prognosis and treatment options.
- The patient and family's knowledge about the meaning of quality of life for their experience.

- Own knowledge of patient and family viewpoints based on relationship and assessment abilities.

Who should I be?

- A courageous nurse who is willing to explore the tensions about the right thing to do.

- A compassionate nurse who is willing to understand the perspectives of all involved.

- A self-confident, self-aware nurse who is accountable and responsible for his or her own knowledge base.

What should I do?

- Verify understanding of patient and family's preferences.

- Ask physician to explain benefits and burdens of treatment.

- Refer to spiritual advisor or psychologist if complexity of situation indicates need for consultation.

- Talk with physician about your understanding of the situation from the patient's perspective.

- Suggest a health team conference or referral to ethics committee to make sure all viewpoints are expressed and understood.

Conflict With Family

A Norwegian nurse who worked in a geriatric unit in a hospital described a conflict between what family members wanted and what the expert knowledge of health professionals indicated was best for the patient.

> *Staff reported frustrations about the patient—should the patient eat? Could she eat? Should she have fluids or not? Was she dying or not? She'd had a stroke and then had problems with swallowing. We were afraid she would get pneumonia, so she didn't get any food. The family wanted to give her food. ... So this was extremely difficult for both the family and for us. I don't know if we solved it very well, but I remember that we had to have a lot of dialogue with the family. I think what was most difficult was for them to stop giving her food. ... But before she died, we allowed the family to give her some small portions of food—not for her, but for them. Like a last wish.*

This nurse also spoke about the need to protect the family from a decision they might regret.

> *We are conscious about not letting them [the family] think that they made the decision. Even if we could agree with them in some parts, we had to let it be our responsibility and then inform them. It's important to have dialogue, but never let them believe that they made the decision. It's important because it would be very hard for the family to think it was the wrong decision. The family shouldn't feel they have to say yes or no. But they should be informed; they should be involved in the discussion in a careful way, but not get this feeling they said "no" and should have said "yes."*

Ethical Conflicts

Autonomy is a significant value in a medical model of care. Patients have the right to make their own decisions. Significant conflicts arise, however, when a patient can no longer make those decisions. Nurses are often in the middle, charged with advocating for the patient but facing decisions that might be in contrast to the patient's wishes. An American palliative care nurse tells of meeting with family members who did not want to honor their mother's health care directive.

> *The patient's health care directive was eloquent. She said that dying was a part of life. She was no longer alert and not able to make decisions. What do you do? Tube feedings? I pulled the three daughters and the son-in-law together. One of the daughters said, "You have to put a feeding tube in, or she'll starve and we'll be killing her." I read the directive out loud to the family. It very clearly delineated no CPR and no artificial feeding. The patient said in her directive, "I don't know what I might be dealing with, but I don't want to be resuscitated and no feeding tube. Look at my quality of life; I'm okay and ready to go. These are tough decisions, but I am taking the burden from you." I told the family that we would not put in a feeding tube because it was against her wishes. It would be unethical and illegal. I turned to the daughter and said, "I'll get the priest. I'll get you the support you need, and we'll keep her comfortable." She died the next day. That daughter was not particularly happy, but we honored her mother's wishes.*
>
> *I usually try to bring in the directive and say, "This meeting is about what your dad wanted, and he can't speak." I say, "If he could speak, what would he say?" Families sometimes say, "Well he'd say forget this."*

While the American nurse advocated for honoring the patient's wishes, she also kept the needs of the family in mind. In this situation, she offered support to the daughter who was struggling with the decision not to place the feeding tube.

Key Points

- Conflicts often arise when caring for patients at the end of life. They can occur between patient and family members, between health care team members, and between patient-family and health care team.

- Nurses have a significant role in addressing conflict because of a holistic approach to the patient.

- Conflicts with patients and families often center on lack of information, lack of consensus about care and treatment, and a breakdown in communication either with other family members or the health care team.

- Ethical conflict is often the result of uncertainty about the right course of action and who should decide.

- Conflict resolution starts with providing accurate and understandable information and eliciting the patient and family's understanding of the situation.

- Reflective practice includes stepping back when a conflict arises and asking

  - Do I understand the other (health care professional, patient-family, physician) point of view?

  - How are my actions, values, and beliefs contributing to the conflict?

  - How can I use this as an opportunity to learn, grow, and become more self-aware?

REFLECTION QUESTIONS

1. Think of a situation where you did not agree with the care a patient was receiving. What did you do? Using information from this chapter, what would you do differently?

2. Analyze a conflict in end-of-life care that you have observed or experienced. Was the conflict effectively resolved? What were the consequences or outcomes of resolving or not resolving the conflict?

3. What are strategies or approaches that can be used to create a unit or organizational environment that reduces the incidence of conflict and moves toward early resolution of conflict?

References

Abbott, K. H., Sago, J. G., Breen, C. M., Abernethy, A. P., & Tulsky, J. A. (2001). Families looking back: One year after discussion of withdrawal or withholding of life-sustaining support. *Critical Care Medicine, 29*, 197-201.

American Medical Association. (1999). *The education for physicians on end of life care (EPEC) curriculum.* The EPEC Project, 1999. Available at http://epec.net

Asch-Goodkin, J. (2000). The virtues of hospice. *Patient Care for the Nurse Practitioner, 3*, 6-18.

Badger, J. M. (2005). A descriptive study of coping strategies used by medical intensive care unit nurses during transitions from cure- to comfort-oriented care. *Heart & Lung, 34*(10), 63-68.

Bolmsjo, I., & Hermeren, G. (2003). Conflicts of interest: Experiences of close relatives of patients suffering from amyotrophic lateral sclerosis. *Nursing Ethics, 10*(2), 187-198.

Bowman, K. (2000a). Communication, negotiation, and mediation: Dealing with conflict in end-of-life decisions. *Journal of Palliative Care, 16*(Suppl.), S17-S23.

Bowman, K. (2000b). *Ian Anderson Continuing Education Program in End-of-Life Care. Module 9: Conflict Resolution.* Continuing Education and the Joint Centre for Bioethics, University of Toronto and the Temmy Latner Centre For Palliative Care, Mount Sinai Hospital. Retrieved July 8, 2008, from http://www.cme.utoronto.ca/endoflife/Modules.htm

Boyle, D. K., Miller, P. A., & Forbes-Thompson, S. A. (2005). Communication and end-of-life care in the intensive care unit: Patient, family, and clinician outcomes. *Critical Care Nursing Quarterly, 28*(4), 302-316.

Breen, C. M., Abernethy A. P., Abbott, K. H., & Tulsky, J. A. (2001). Conflict associated with decisions to limit life-sustaining treatment in intensive care units. *Journal of General Internal Medicine, 16*, 401-415.

Breier-Mackie, S. (2001). Patient autonomy and medical paternity: Can nurses help doctors listen to patients? *Nursing Ethics, 8*(6), 510-521.

Buchanan, S. F., Desrochers, J. M., Henry, D. B., Thomassen, G., & Barrett, Jr., P. H. (2002). A mediation/medical advisory panel model for resolving disputes about end-of-life care. *The Journal of Clinical Ethics, 13*(3), 188-202.

Burt, R. A. (2002). The medical futility debate: Patient choice, physician obligation, and end-of-life care. *Journal of Palliative Medicine, 5*(2), 249-252.

Cameron, M. E. (1993). *Living with AIDS: Experiencing ethical problems.* Newbury Park, CA: Sage.

Dahlin, C. M., & Gianiracusa, D. E. (2006). Communication in palliative care. In B. R. Ferrell & N. Coyle (Eds.). *Textbook of palliative nursing* (pp. 67-93). New York: Oxford University Press.

Dawson, K. A. (2008). Palliative care for critically ill older adults: Dimensions of nursing advocacy. *Critical Care Nursing Quarterly, 31*(1), 19-23.

Elpern, E. H., Covert, B., & Kleinpell, R. (2005). Moral distress of staff nurses on a medical intensive care unit. *American Journal of Critical Care, 14*(6), 523-530.

Enes, S. P. D. & de Vries. (2004). A survey of ethical issues experienced by nurses caring for terminally ill elderly people. *Nursing Ethics, 11*(2), 25-264.

Ferrand, E., Lemaire, F., Regnier, B., Kuteifan, K., Badet, M., Asfar, P., et al. (2003). Discrepancies between perceptions by physicians and nursing staff of intensive care unit end-of-life decisions. *American Journal of Respiratory and Critical Care Medicine, 167*, 1310-1315.

Hsieh, H., Shannon, S. E., & Curtis, J. R. (2006). Contradictions and communication strategies during end-of-life decision making in the intensive care unit. *Journal of Critical Care, 21*, 294-304.

Jezuit, D. L. (2000). Suffering of critical care nurses with end-of-life decisions. *MEDSURG Nursing, 9*(3), 145-152.

Kendall, A., & Arnold, R. (n.d.). *Fast fact and concept #183: Conflict resolution I: Careful communication.* American Academy of Hospice and Palliative Medicine. Retrieved July 8, 2008, from http://www.aahpm.org/cgi-bin/wkcgi/view?status=A%20&search=145&id=706&offset=250&limit=25

Kendall, A., & Arnold, R. (n.d). *Fast fact and concept #184: Conflict resolution II: Principled negotiation.* American Academy of Hospice and Palliative Medicine. Retrieved July 8, 2008, from http://www.aahpm.org/cgi-bin/wkcgi/view?status=A%20&search=145&id=707&offset=250&limit=25

Ladd, R. E., Pasquella, L., & Smith, S. (2000). What to do when the end is near: Ethical issues in home care nursing. *Public Health Nursing, 17*(2), 103-110.

Mari, C., Farrell, C. A., Lacroix, J., Graeme, R., & Shemie, S. D. (2000). Decision making and end-of-life care in critically ill children. *Journal of Palliative Care, 16* (Suppl.), S45-S52.

Miller, C., Funk, & Wiegand, D. (2006). Judgments of nurses and physicians regarding futility and withdrawal of treatment in medical and surgical intensive care units (ICUs). *American Journal of Critical Care, 15*(3), 326-327.

Oberle, K. (2001). Doctors' and nurses' perceptions of ethical problems in end-of-life decisions. *Journal of Advanced Nursing, 33*(6), 707-715.

Pattison, N. (2004). Integration of critical care and palliative care at the end of life. *British Journal of Nursing, 13*(3), 132-139.

Robertson, D. W. (1996). Ethical theory, ethnography, and differences between doctors and nurses in approaches to patient care. *Journal of Medical Ethics, 22*, 292-299.

Rushton, C. H. (1992). Care-giver suffering in critical care nursing. *Heart & Lung, 21*(3), 303-306.

Rushton, C. H., Williams, M. A., & Sabatier, K. H. (2002). The integration of palliative care and critical care: One vision, one voice. *Critical Care Nursing Clinics of North America, 14*, 133-140.

Schaffer, M. A. (2007). Ethical problems in end-of-life decisions for elderly Norwegians. *Nursing Ethics, 14*(2), 242-257.

Stanley, K. J., & Zoloth-Dorfman, L. (2006). Ethical considerations in B. R. Ferrell & N. Coyle (Eds.), *Textbook of palliative nursing* (pp. 1031-1053). New York: Oxford University Press.

The, A. M., Hak, T., Koeter, G., & van der Wal, G. (2000). Collusion in doctor-patient communication about imminent death: An ethnographic study. *British Medical Journal, 321*(7273), 1376-1381.

Weaver, A. W. (2004). Family health promotion during life-threatening illness at the end of life. In P. T. Bomar (Ed.), *Promoting health in families: Applying family research and theory to nursing practice* (pp. 507-533). Philadelphia: Saunders.

Zuzelo, P. R. (2007). Exploring the moral distress of registered nurses. *Nursing Ethics, 14*(3), 344-359.

We were looking at ways to improve pain relief for our patients on the oncology unit. Did we need to educate the nurses? Work with the doctors? So, we tracked the amount of time it took from when the patient said he had pain to when he got medication. What we discovered was that it took a long time, and it wasn't because of one player. When the nurse assessed the pain, she had to contact the doctor, the doctor had to write the orders, the orders had to go to the pharmacy, the pharmacy had several steps they had to take, and so forth. In order to ensure that the patient got prompt pain relief, we had to change the whole system. And it had to be a team effort— nurses, doctors, pharmacists, and administrators all working together. I believe that we did it because nurses took the lead.

—Oncology nurse manager

6

·

Advocating: When Nurses Need to Take Action

Advocacy is an essential skill for nurses as we care for our dying patients. It means listening to our patients and speaking on their behalf at the bedside, and it means looking at our systems and whether they "work" on behalf of our patients. Patients who are nearing the end of life are vulnerable, and that often places them in situations that require immediate action. The overall goal of advocacy is to provide care that is of the greatest benefit to the patient (Jezuit, 2000).

What Is Advocacy?

Thacker (2008) identified four defining characteristics of advocacy based on a literature review that was focused on advocacy in professional practice:

1. protecting the patient,

2. listening to the patient's voice,

3. making moral and ethical decisions, and

4. promoting well-being.

For nurses, the advocacy role is about providing support for what patients want or need for their well-being. In a qualitative study of 24 military nurses on their perceptions of the meaning of advocacy, the analysis resulted in an overall theme of "safeguarding" with additional subthemes of protecting, attending, being the patient's voice, and preserving the patient's identity (Foley, Minick, & Key, 2000). Sorensen and Iedema (2007) categorized three advocacy themes or concepts in the literature specific to end-of-life care situations:

1. protection of patients against medical treatment they do not want,

2. removing discomfort resulting from unnecessary treatment so the patient can die in peace, and

3. empowerment of patients through increasing their awareness of patients' rights to assist them in making informed decisions.

Tschudin and Hunt (1994) suggested that three elements must be present for the nursing advocacy role:

1. being proactive rather than passive,

2. speaking up and acting on behalf of the patient, and

3. a conflict or problem that necessitates an advocacy action.

In addition, the recognition of vulnerability in an unjust situation, along with a feeling of a sense of responsibility to respond to the situation, leads to a response of advocacy (Spenceley, Reuter, & Allen, 2006).

McSteen and Peden-McAlpine (2006) analyzed the stories of seven nurses who experienced ethical challenges and believed they acted as an advocate for dying patients. They identified three subplots or themes with related advocacy activities that were common among the experiences of all seven nurses:

1. acting as a guide during transition at the end of life (providing and clarifying information),

2. acting as a liaison between the health care team and family (linking with the health care team to help all understand goals and plan of care), and

3. acting to support the meaning of the illness to patients and families (affirming the choices that patients and families made according to their values and goals, which may not be consistent with nurses' beliefs of what should be done).

Advocacy Definitions

An Advocate:

- "Pleads someone else's cause or acts on someone else's behalf, with a focus on developing the community, system, individual, or family's capacity to plead their own cause or on their own behalf" (Minnesota Department of Health, 2001, p. 263).

- Assists patients and families to overcome barriers impeding the care path (Wilkie, 2001).

- Informs a patient of options and supports whatever decision a patient makes (Kohnke, 1982).

- Takes "explicit actions" to represent the wishes of patients in matters related to their dying and death in health care institutions" (Gillon, 1986, in Sorenson & Iedema, 2007, p. 1344).

- Takes "knowledge-based" action intended to improve health by influencing system-level decisions; political advocacy (Spenceley, Reutter, & Allen, 2006, p. 184).

Advocacy Outcomes

In a thorough analysis of the literature, Thacker (2008) identified the following outcomes for patient and family that result from advocacy actions by nurses:

- safe care,

- improved quality of life,

- patient autonomy and self-determination,

- patient and family education,

- dignity of life, and

- comfort and minimal suffering.

For nurses, outcomes included work satisfaction and their own empowerment in the practice of advocacy.

Barriers and Supports to Advocacy Action

Being an advocate is more complicated than simply implementing advocacy actions. Complex health care environments with many "players" contain barriers that can interfere with follow-through on advocacy actions. In a study with a sample of 317 nurses, Thacker (2008) found the three most frequent barriers experienced in practicing advocacy in end-of-life nursing care were

1. physicians,

2. patients' families, and

3. fear.

"Although all sources of knowledge are important and relevant—nursing knowledge, medical knowledge, and patient knowledge—the capacity to act is often forestalled by hierarchical relationships."

Other barriers to advocating for the dying include nursing characteristics such as negative attitudes toward death, lack of skills needed to care for dying patients, a sense of the importance of maintaining professional distance, and having a task orientation that does not include the communication aspects of end-of-life care.

System characteristics also dampen attempts at advocacy, including a hierarchical structure that gives more power to physicians, and an oppressive unit or organizational culture. When advocating for patients, nurses may risk being caught in the middle, leading to conflict and moral distress. In some situations, advocacy actions could put the nurse's job at risk (Copp, 1994; Pimple & Schmidt, 2001; Thacker, 2006, 2008).

Differences in professional power can lead to ineffectiveness in advocacy actions for nurses. In patriarchal systems, it is possible to actually lose sight of patients' rights (Thacker, 2008). Although all sources of knowledge are important and relevant—nursing knowledge, medical knowledge, and patient knowledge—the capacity to act is often forestalled by hierarchical relationships (Sorensen & Iedema, 2007). In their ethnographic study of an intensive care unit, Sorensen and Iedema concluded that although nurses reported physicians' attitudes were a barrier to implementing advocacy actions, the nurses also did not work together to challenge the physicians' approaches or find other ways of interacting with physicians that would reduce a sense of powerlessness. The nurses were not advocating for the nursing profession.

Thacker (2008) found nurses did experience support in their advocacy actions. Support for nurses' advocacy role in the beginning, experienced, and expert levels of practice came from their nurse managers and co-workers; from working in multidisciplinary teams; from their relationships with patients and families; and from their own knowledge, beliefs, and compassion.

Advocacy Models

Models of advocacy provide a way to understand why advocacy is important and how it is done. These models also indicate how aspects of systems may intensify the need for advocacy. Advocacy is needed when something is wrong with the system, whether it is a health care institution process or structure or other societal process or structure that allows for taking advantage of or ignoring vulnerability. Advocacy can be understood as a process, closely paralleling the nursing process (Minnesota Department of Health, 2001). A step-by-step process is a systematic approach to advocacy action.

Basic Steps for Advocacy

- Assess the nature and source of the issues to be addressed.
- Determine the appropriate "target" for the advocacy intervention.
- Establish objectives with the patient.
- Negotiate the action plan with a patient, family, group, system, or community. The plan must indicate the clients' capacity to speak or act on their own behalf and the assistance they desire.
- Determine resource availability.
- Assess to what extent the advocacy "target" may be receptive, and adjust the action plan accordingly.
- Implement.
- Evaluate.

Source: Minnesota Department of Health, 2001, p. 265

Fowler (1989) identified four conceptual models useful to nurses in their advocacy role. The model or approach used will depend on the purpose of the advocacy action.

1. The nurse is a protector of rights and, as a professional, is qualified to plead the cause of the patient in the context of the health care team (Spenceley et al., 2006).

2. The nurse is a preserver of values by focusing on empowering patients to act based on their values; this is a form of "decisional counseling" (Fowler, 1989).

3. The nurse is a defender of persons; it is morally right to support the needs and rights of others, which is connected to human rights rather than legal rights (Spenceley et al., 2006).

4. The nurse is a champion of social justice and addresses the inequities inherent in health care. In addition to meeting the needs of individuals and families, the nurse also is involved in upstream advocacy "intended to influence change in the structures and relationships that contribute to the poor health of groups and populations" (Spenceley et al., 2006, p. 182). In the situation of end-of-life care, advocacy is intended to change systems that contribute to poor dying experiences for patients and population groups.

Advocacy Skills

A broad base of skills is required to fulfill the advocacy role effectively. At a basic level, advocacy is about providing good nursing care. Interpersonal communication skills are needed, as well as communication skills necessary to advocate effectively with health professionals and organizational systems for the needs of dying persons and their families. The nurse needs a repertoire of sound clinical judgment, sensitive caring practices, collaborative skills, systems thinking, and commitment to inquiry about best practices (Rushton, Williams, & Sabatier, 2002). See sidebar, "Advocacy Skills in Providing End-of-Life Care," for an extensive list of useful advocacy skills for nurses who provide end-of-life care. In advocacy, nurses will serve the patient's best interests by presenting a realistic picture of the patient's situation to the patient, family, and health care team members. By doing so, decisions can be made based on the best evidence available, including evidence about the patient as a person. A realistic picture of the patient's situation is not always easily heard or accepted, but paying attention to what is really happening regarding the patient's status and prognosis will ultimately reduce suffering and result in better care for the patient.

Advocacy Skills in Providing End-of-Life Care

Advocacy in Patient Care

- Anticipate effects of illness progression and side effects of medications.
- Reassure patient and family that future problems will be attended to.
- Work with health care team to identify most effective pharmacological and nonpharmacological interventions.
- Consult with physician on management of difficult symptoms.
- Reinforce and support patient's decisions.
- Present a realistic picture of the patient as a person to the health care team.

Advocacy for Families

- Assist in finding resources for resolving conflict, clarifying goals, and follow-up to make sure family's needs are being met.
- Help family members "reframe" the patient's situation so they are realistic about expectations.

Advocacy in Situations of Diversity

- Examine actions to make sure your values are not negatively affecting what is best for the patient.
- Avoid cultural stereotyping and generalizations by being aware that differences *within* groups are often greater than those *among* groups.

Characteristics of Advocacy Actions

- Be assertive: Do not take "no" as the final answer.
- Be willing to take risks, but consider whether you are bending or breaking a rule.
- Negotiate with the goal of creating a "win-win" situation.
- Stretch beyond your comfort zone to find new ways of understanding and influencing.
- Collaborate with others who are "like-minded."

Important Nursing Virtues

- Trustworthiness: Build trusting relationships with patients and families.

- Compassion: Reassure patients that their suffering matters to others and deserves a response.

- Courage: Help initiate advocacy action in a situation that may not be supported by others within the system.

- Prudence: Know when action will move toward change, will not lead to change, or will cause harm.

Sources: Egan, 1998; Jezuit, 2000; McSteen & Peden-McApline, 2006; Minnesota Department of Health, 2001; Robichaux & Park, 2006; Stanley & Zoloth-Dorfman, 2006.

Advocacy in Specific End-of-Life Situations

Advance Care Planning

An important area for nursing advocacy is in advance care planning. Prolonging the dying process increases suffering for patients and contributes to the moral distress of nurses who care for them. Both the physical suffering of patients and moral distress of nurses can be mitigated through advance care planning. The Respecting Patient Choices Program (RPCP) in Australia was designed to educate nurses for the consultant role in advance care planning with patients (Seal, 2007). Nurses participated in a 2-day course that included a focus on patient advocacy and systemic support for a good death. In a randomized, controlled trial, 84% of the nurses who received the advocacy training indicated their work environment supported helping patients understand and make informed choices about treatments, in comparison with 49% of the control group. In addition, fewer nurses in the educated group felt powerless to advocate for patients for appropriate end-of-life care. The comments of two nurses in a follow-up focus group indicate a move toward a culture change as a result of participation in RPCP:

> "I think it changes the whole culture about what we are doing."

> "Since having the RPCP, a lot more care and respect is given to end-stage patients" (Seal, 2007, p. 34).

Residential Facilities for Elderly

In another Australian study, investigators explored the perceptions and beliefs about palliative care of 60 nurses and care assistants who worked in residential care facilities for elderly patients. Advocacy as a key role was one of the themes identified from an analysis of the focus group data (Phillips et al., 2006). The participants made the following points about their experience with advocacy-related work:

1. Participants believed it was their responsibility to follow through with residents' requests for end-of-life care; however, they found it difficult to make that happen when a resident was transferred to a hospital, which sometimes occurred when family members or the physician wanted the transfer but the patient did not.

2. Transfer occurred more often in situations in which there was family tension or lack of agreement on what to do.

3. Participants believed transfer to the hospital was disorienting for residents and resulted in more invasive procedures; they also indicated families were frequently unrealistic about what could be accomplished in acute intervention and expected that care would be better in the hospital than in the residential facility.

4. For participants, the advocacy role meant giving patients and families more information about likely outcomes of additional interventions, so that their decisions would be informed decisions.

Provision of Aggressive Care

Robichaux and Clark (2006) interviewed 21 U.S.-based, expert critical care nurses about the ethical dilemma of providing aggressive care that would not result in an acceptable quality of life for the patient. Two of three themes resulting from the analysis directly relate to advocacy—protecting or speaking to the patient, and presenting a realistic picture. For vulnerable patients, the nurses believed that family members did not understand the consequences and difficulties associated with treatment, and this lack of understanding delayed the reframing of expectations for recovery. Nurses believed they should clarify for the family how the patient would experience the interventions. The third theme, experiencing frustration and resignation, is actually a barrier to advocacy.

Advocacy for a Palliative Care Approach

Advocacy for end-of-life patients and their families will become easier as palliative care approaches are integrated into critical care and other relevant settings. Sorensen and Iedema (2007) suggest advocacy efforts be focused beyond the defense of patients' rights to a focus on political advocacy. In a nutshell, they argue that we need to advocate for the nursing profession to remove the barriers that make nurses less likely to carry out advocacy actions.

"Courage, compassion, and intuition can lead us into advocacy, but we also need advocacy skills and collective action in order to change the status quo that has indicated treatment and cure over comfort, holistic care, and healing at the end of life."

Spenceley et al. (2006) suggest that for nurses to be more influential in advocating at the policy level, several challenges inherent in the practice context need to be addressed. For one, workforce issues such as understaffing, powerlessness in organizations, and lack of time available to nurses need to be resolved, because it takes time and energy to initiate collaboration for change. In addition, socialization to the profession is more often consistent with avoiding risk and encourages conformity or even silence in situations of conflict or confrontation. This means changing norms of the profession (Anna, 1995), so that we are willing to take action by making sure our advocacy "voice" is not only shared, but also heard. Nurses can put forth their nursing knowledge and advocate for patients so that their patient knowledge is also heard.

System-Oriented Advocacy Actions in End-of-Life Care

- Define the advocacy role for the profession of nursing.

- Promote acceptance of the nursing advocacy role by nurses, patients, families, and other health professionals.

- Challenge personal assumptions about lack of power and seek to change hierarchical structures that devalue the contributions of nurses.

- Negotiate differences in attitudes, values, and end-of-life care practices with other professionals.

- Develop and promote implementation of a comfort-care plan.

- Increase the percentage of terminally ill patients who are discharged to home hospice care.

- Encourage the practice of timelier end-of-life decisions early in the hospital admission of terminally ill clients.

- Ensure that nursing education contains substantial content and process on nursing roles in advocacy and policy development, as well as content on high-quality end-of-life care.

- Initiate collaborative interdisciplinary and disciplinary approaches that are focused on improvement of end-of-life care.

- Unify voices through partnerships—the Hospice and Palliative Care Coalition is a partnership of the following organizations:

    - Hospice and Palliative Nurses Association

    - American Academy of Hospice and Palliative Medicine

    - National Hospice and Palliative Care Organization

Sources: Fins et al., 1999; Scanlon, 2006; Sorenson & Iedema, 2007; Spenceley et al., 2006.

Both collaboration and coalition building can make advocacy more powerful and reach more people and organizations. In collaboration, two or more people or organizations work to achieve a common goal. See sidebar, "Basic Steps of Collaboration." Collaboration is needed to facilitate a "lane change," which is the "shift in thinking from acute treatment aimed at cure to one that is focused on the active palliation of symptoms and the preparation for death and bereavement" (Thompson, McClement, & Daeninck, 2006, p. 92).

System factors that need to be addressed to facilitate a lane change are the absence of a unit philosophy of palliative care and the differences in palliative care approaches between nurses and physicians—holistic care versus an emphasis on cure. Nurses can initiate collaborative processes through a committee or task force to work toward a unit philosophy of palliative care and then engage physician leadership to discuss how both disciplines can work together to provide quality end-of-life care for patients and families.

Basic Steps of Collaboration

- Convene or join the collaborative group.
- Select a structure (ad hoc, informal or formal, open or closed membership).
- Determine leadership selection process.
- Structure decision-making process (consensus, majority rule).
- Identify collaborative actions (advocacy in this case).
- Develop the plan.
- Decrease barriers to collaborative action (e.g., avoid turf issues, make communication a priority, develop clear rules).
- Evaluate results.

Source: Minnesota Department of Health, 2001, pp. 180-182.

Coalition building is similar to collaboration because it involves collective action, but there is a greater focus on bringing in outside organizations. Collaborative initiatives usually stay within an organization or community. Coalition building promotes and develops "alliances among organizations or constituencies for a common purpose. With coalition building, one can develop linkages, solve problems, and enhance local leadership to address health concerns" (Minnesota Department of Health, 2001, p. 211). See sidebar, "Basic Steps of Coalition Building." An example of a coalition is the Hospice and Palliative Care Coalition, which is a partnership of the Hospice and Palliative Nurses Association, the American Academy of Hospice and Palliative Medicine, and the National Hospice and Palliative Care Organization. Together these organizations strengthen the voice for integrating a palliative care approach into acute care and other settings. Coalition builders can develop resources to advocate for quality end-of-life care through publicity, leadership, and promotion of best practices based on research evidence.

Basic Steps of Coalition Building

* Decide to come together.
* Recruit the right members.
* Devise a set of preliminary objectives and activities.
* Convene the coalition.
* Anticipate human, material, and financial resources required to accomplish the goal.
* Select an appropriate structure (short-term or long-term, location and frequency of meetings, membership criteria, decision-making process, agenda setting, and rules for participation).
* Maintain the vitality of the coalition (share power and leadership, anticipate and deal with conflict, provide training, celebrate success).
* Make improvements through evaluation.

Source: Minnesota Department of Health, 2001, pp. 214-217

Reflective Practice

Advocacy skills can be learned, and the practice of advocacy can bring comfort to nurses as well as to patients and their families. Often the easier path is to follow through with the continued treatment that has been chosen by the physician. However, in a medical model that emphasizes aggressive treatment, this path often does not enhance the quality of life but can actually take away quality through causing greater suffering. In this situation, there are many losses. The patient and family can lose the opportunity for more quality time and the experience of a peaceful death. The patient, family, and health care system lose financial resources through unnecessary expenditures. Nurses may lose their integrity as they provide care that seems unnecessary and unwanted.

It is too easy to say we don't have time to engage in dialogue or work toward changing aggressive health care practices at the end of life. But we also need to consider the wear and tear caused by the frustration of providing care for which we do not approve. Our time is much more effective if we use it in intervening to promote a peaceful death in situations where aggressive care is not beneficial or warranted.

We should not blame physicians entirely for the proliferation of unnecessary and unwanted aggressive treatment. We need to look at our own profession of nursing and examine what keeps us silent in situations where we need to speak. The literature indicates the important role of nurses in providing a realistic picture of the end-of-life situation. We can add to our evidence base a knowledge of patient and family perceptions that is enhanced by our day-to-day interactions with them. By bringing quality end-of-life care to the forefront, we can establish the credibility and worth of nursing knowledge. By dialoging with the health care team to focus on best practices for end-of-life care, we can consider the needs and wants of patients and families to fulfill the advocacy role. Courage, compassion, and intuition can lead us into advocacy, but we also need advocacy skills and collective action to change the status quo that has indicated treatment and cure over comfort, holistic care, and healing at the end of life.

Ethical Practice in Advocacy

ETHICAL PROBLEM: What should I do when too many patients are receiving aggressive care at the end of life that is doing little good?

What Should I Value?

- Quality of life.

- The expert knowledge of physicians.

- Effective use of health care resources.

- What patients and their families want.

- Having all voices heard.

Who Should I Be?

- A compassionate nurse who identifies and values what patients and families want.

- A courageous and respectful nurse who is willing to speak up about what patients or families want.

- A skilled nurse who understands how to use processes for effective collaborative work and how to build coalitions.

What Should I Do?

- Gather data about the situation. This could be a survey of nurses or health care team members on their attitudes and values about end-of-life care, or their perceptions of barriers and supports in the health care organization for a palliative care approach.

- Present the findings with recommendations for promoting high quality end-of-life care.

- Form an interdisciplinary task force to develop a leadership plan to facilitate a "lane change" from aggressive treatment at the end of life to a palliative care approach (based on assessment of prognosis).

- Read the evidence on best practices for high quality end-of-life care.

- Join an organization to learn about effective strategies in leading professional change for supporting best practices in high quality end-of-life care.

Nurses' Stories

Assuring Patient Comfort

Nurses are responsible for assuring the comfort and dignity of dying patients. This can be especially challenging in a hospital setting where nurses are working under physicians' orders. A medical-surgical nurse reports how she advocated for a dying patient with a hip fracture:

> I had a patient with end-stage dementia who came in with a hip fracture and [was] in pain. She was yelling, "Help me! Help me!" But I had a doctor who wouldn't write an order for Haldol over 2.5 mg. She said the patient wasn't dying, and a higher dose of Haldol was not appropriate. I said, "I really think she's dying." The doctor wanted to focus on the medical stuff. I did what I could do and explained that I strongly felt the patient was dying. The next day I looked at the chart, and the physician had written hospice care orders. I think she'd thought about it. Sometimes you begin advocating for your patients by planting the seed.

Believing the Patient

Advocacy often begins by listening to our patients and believing what they say. A home care nurse talks about a patient with a long history of mental illness:

> We'd had this patient on and off our home care program many times. She had a history of exaggerating symptoms, and her doctor had labeled her "an attention getter." After a hospitalization for shortness of breath, she was referred back to us. The social worker and I went out to see her and she said, "I don't think I'm doing very well." We could both see that she had changed and that she looked very sick. When we asked the doctor for a referral to hospice, the doctor refused. "She needs to be on her psych meds and she'll be fine." We both disagreed and finally ended up in a heated discussion with the doctor. We said, "We believe the patient is dying, and the patient says she's dying." Reluctantly, the doctor wrote the order for hospice. The patient died 10 days later—at home where she wanted to be.

The key for the nurse in this situation was having the support of her team member, the social worker. Between the two of them, they were able to persist to overcome the physician's reluctance.

Advocating When There Are System Barriers

A Norwegian nurse in a palliative care unit in a nursing home spoke about organizational rules that made it difficult to meet a patient's needs to visit her home and family:

> We have this patient—she was very ill. She had cancer everywhere. She was relatively young. She had a family. Her family was living in the house, and she had a daughter and sons, and some of them were living there too. And she wanted so badly to go home—not to stay home, but to visit them. And she could, but she needed an ambulance. An ambulance is so expensive. . . . I think that it should be so obvious to get. I think she got it, but I think there were rules that restricted her—some rules that said the ambulance cannot be used that way. And we knew she would die soon. She did get home, but I think there were some rules and barriers that made it difficult to work through.

The nurse believed it was a community responsibility to provide ambulance service for this patient so she could get to her home to be with her family. In the interview, the nurse commented that the patient had paid taxes all her life and would get little benefit from her tax money. She reflected that the consequences that result from rules often have more far-reaching effects than intended. In this situation, the rules about the use of the ambulance were in the way of effective end-of-life care for the patient.

Key Points

* Nurse advocacy for patients at the end of life is a skill that can be learned. It takes place with individual patients and families, health care team members (including physicians), as well as with systems.

- Nursing advocacy includes acting on the patient's behalf, protecting the patient from unwanted care and treatment, promoting patient well-being, and assisting with moral and ethical decision-making.

- Advocacy by nurses results in improved quality of life, patient autonomy, patient and family knowledge, and affirmation of patient/family values and beliefs.

- Barriers to advocacy action include a hierarchical health care structure that results in disempowerment of the nursing profession, lack of support from other nurses, and a complex, often bewildering health care environment.

- Advocacy is a process similar to the nursing process that involves assessing the nature of the issues, establishing goals with the patient/family, identifying key players, establishing a plan, and evaluating that plan.

- Collaboration and coalition building are important aspects of advocacy when creating and implementing systems changes that will improve end-of-life care.

REFLECTION QUESTIONS

1. Think of the health care organization where you are now working or where you previously worked. Analyze the barriers and supports for nursing advocacy actions for dying patients.

2. Using one of the nursing stories above, analyze how you would apply the basic steps for advocacy to implement advocacy action.

3. Reflect on what advocacy skills you would like to develop and what you need to do to become more skilled in advocacy for dying patients and their families.

References

Anna, G. J. (1995). How we lie. *Hastings Center Report, 26*(Suppl.), S12-S14.

Copp, C. (1994). Palliative care nursing education: A review of research findings. *Journal of Advanced Nursing, 19*, 552-557.

Egan, G. (1998). *The skilled helper: A problem-management approach to helping.* Pacific Grove: Brooks-Cole.

Fins, J. J., Miller, F. G., Acres, C. A., Bacchetta, M. D., Hazzard, L. L, & Raplcin, D. D. (1999). End of life decision making in the hospital: Current practice and future prospects. *Journal of Pain and Symptom Management, 17*(1), 6-15.

Foley, B. J., Minick, P., & Kee, C. (2000). Nursing advocacy during a military operation. *Western Journal of Nursing Research, 22*, 492-507.

Fowler, D. M. (1989). Social advocacy: Ethical issues in critical care. *Heart & Lung, 18*(1), 97-99.

Gillon, R. (1986). Nursing ethics and medical ethics. *Journal of Medical Ethics, 22*(1), 115-116.

Jezuit, D. L. (2000). Suffering of critical care nurses with end-of-life decisions. *MEDSURG Nursing, 9*(3), 145-152.

Kohnke, M. F. (1982). *Advocacy: Risk and reality.* St. Louis, MO: CV Mosby.

McSteen, K., & Peden-McAlpine, C. (2006). The role of the nurse as advocate in ethically difficult care situations with dying patients. *Journal of Hospice and Palliative Nursing, 8*(5), 259-269.

Minnesota Department of Health, Public Health Nursing Section. (2001). *Public health interventions—Applications for public health nursing practice.* St. Paul, MN: Author.

Phillips, J., Davidson, P. M., Jackson, D., Kristjanson, L., Daly, J., & Curran, J. (2006). Residential aged care: The last frontier for palliative care. *Journal of Advanced Nursing, 55*(4), 416-424.

Pimple, C., & Schmidt, L. (2001). Nursing education: Advocating for the dying. *The Kansas Nurse, 76*(7), 8-12.

Robichaux, C., & Clark, A. P. (2006). Practice of expert critical care nurses in situations of prognostic conflict at the end of life. *American Journal of Critical Care, 15*(5), 480-489.

Rushton, C. H., Williams, M. A., & Sabatier, K. H. (2002). The integration of palliative care in critical care: One vision, one voice. *Critical Care Nursing Clinics of North America, 14*, 133-140.

Scanlon, C. (2006). Public policy and end-of-life care: The nurse's role. In B. R. Ferrell & N. Coyle (Eds.), *Textbook of palliative nursing* (pp. 1055-1066). New York: Oxford University Press.

Seal, M. (2007). Patient advocacy and advance care planning in the acute hospital setting. *Australian Journal of Advanced Nursing*, *24*(4), 29-36.

Sorenson, R., & Iedema, R. (2007). Advocacy at the end of life: Research design: An ethnographic study of an ICU. *International Journal of Nursing Studies*, *44*, 1343-1353.

Spenceley, S. M., Reuter, L., & Allen, M. N. (2006). The road less traveled: Nursing advocacy at the policy level. *Policy, Politics, & Nursing Practice*, *7*(3), 180-194.

Stanley, K. J. & Zoloth-Dorfman, L. (2006). Ethical considerations. In B. R. Ferrell & N. Coyle (Eds.), *Textbook of palliative nursing* (pp. 1031-1053.). New York: Oxford University Press.

Thacker, K. S. (2006). *The perceptions of advocacy behaviors in end-of-life nursing care among novice, experienced and expert nurses.* Unpublished Dissertation, Widener University School of Nursing, Chester, Pennsylvania.

Thacker, K. S. (2008). Nurses' advocacy behaviors in end-of-life nursing care. *Nursing Ethics*, *15*(2), 174-185.

Thompson, G. N, McClement, S. E., & Daeninck, P. J. (2006). Changing lanes: Facilitating the transition from curative to palliative care. *Journal of Palliative Care*, *22*(2), 91-98.

Tschudin, V., & Hunt, G. (1994). Moving into a new era. *Nursing Ethics*, *1*(1), 1-2.

Wilkie, D. J. (2001). *Toolkit for nursing excellence at end-of-life transition* [CD-ROM]. Seattle, WA: University of Washington School of Nursing.

I had this aunt who lived her last years in a nursing home. I didn't get to see her much because of the distance. She died in the nursing home, and I didn't get there until the next day. I walked into her empty room. There was a nurse sitting on the bed crying. She told me how much my aunt meant to her. I was so comforted knowing that someone cared about her.

–Retired Nurse

7

·

Saying Goodbye at the End of Life

For dying patients and their families, the nurse is often the closest resource they have for help in saying goodbye. We can provide the clinical expertise to help make the dying process comfortable and peaceful. More importantly, we can provide the presence and sometimes the words to promote a safe transition. Whether the death is a sudden event or the end of a long journey, nurses are key to assuring a peaceful life completion.

Your Role in Saying Goodbye

Saying goodbye to someone who is dying can influence how family members adjust and look to the future. Dying patients identify the importance of maintaining close personal relationships. For some, this means being surrounded by family; for others, it means the healing of difficult relationships. Prince-Paul (2008) noted that, "Nurses have the opportunity to lay the groundwork for addressing the meaning of close personal relationships, their importance, and how the importance of the relationship is communicated" (p. 370).

In studies focused on the needs of family caregivers of dying patients, communication and the need for information were two of the most important concerns identified. Furthermore, caregivers expressed relief at being able to talk about the impending death of their family member with nurses (Lowrey, 2008).

Lassig (2008) suggests using "gentle guidance" in encouraging family members to plan a time to say important things or write a letter to their terminally ill family member. Saying goodbye should be an intentional process. In a study of 28 bereaved individuals on the meaning and processes of saying goodbye, all but one spoke about saying goodbye to their loved one before death (Lassig). Saying goodbye had relational and spatial-based meanings as well as final acts of connectedness. Study participants wanted to be physically close to the dying person and took steps to reduce physical distance, including lying in the bed with the patient. Final acts of connectedness included taking trips, sharing last words, giving advice, writing letters, and planning funerals. Some participants stayed awake all night so that they could be near the dying person.

An understanding of what patients and families want in their final communications can help guide what nurses suggest to patients and families about how to say goodbye. Keeley (2007) sampled individuals who had experienced final conversations with loved ones. The most common message conveyed was an expression of love. Other messages were about identity, religion and spirituality, routine and everyday content, and difficult relationship issues. Byock (2004) suggested specific phrases family members can use when saying goodbye, including "thank you" and "I love you." Additionally, phrases such as "we will miss you" and "now you can have peace" may provide comfort for both family members and the dying patient (Poor & Gary, 2001). Norlander (2008) notes that nurses can provide guidance to families in saying goodbye with concrete tasks:

- teaching caregiving functions such as skin care, gentle massage, or turning and positioning;

- encouraging family story-telling; and

- encouraging family rituals such as singing favorite songs, reciting familiar prayers, or reading from favorite books.

When the dying person is unresponsive, remind family members that their loved one may hear what is being said. It may also be helpful for family members to give permission for the person to die and say that those left behind will be all right (Poor & Gary, 2001). The Center on Aging (2004) at the John A. Burns School of Medicine suggests dying people need to be assured of five things:

1. their responsibilities will be taken care of,

2. the survivors will continue life without them,

3. all is forgiven,

4. their life was meaningful, and

5. they will be remembered.

Be aware that patients and families come from a variety of cultural and religious backgrounds. (See Chapter 8.) Avoid using clichés such as "He's in the hands of God" or "The Lord never gives us more than we can handle" (Norlander, 2008).

Letting Go

For dying people, letting go is a gradual process of transitioning from a life based in the physical world and within social relationships to a few key relationships and, finally, to an inner focus (Egan & Labyak, 2006). Letting go requires accepting the reality of the terminally ill diagnosis. It involves cognitive and emotional work. One researcher explored the concept of letting go in family decisions to forgo life support for a critically ill family member (Swigart, Lidz, Butterworth, & Arnold, 1996). Those family members who were able to make the decision to forgo life support had worked through understanding and reframing the illness, reviewing and revising the dying person's life story, and had continued their family roles and relationships. Family members realized that recovery was not likely, experienced a sense of continuity in life processes, and were confident relationships would be intact. In the process of working through accepting and anticipating death, family members reframed the patient's life story to include death and reflected on how the death of the family member would affect their own lives (Swigart et al., 1996).

When health professionals focus on medical care, they may overlook the work that family members need to go through to reframe the situation so that they can let go.

All those involved may be at various places in the process of letting go. When health professionals focus on medical care, they may overlook the work that family members need to go through to reframe the situation so that they can let go. Family members and patients view situations from their total life experiences and want the dying person to be well and continue their life, while health professionals more often focus closely on the critical illness (Swigart et al., 1996). Because of these different perspectives, as well as the hectic pace of the health care environment, it is challenging for health professionals to pay attention to the letting go process experienced by those dying and their family members. Nurses need to be aware of and facilitate processes that can help family members let go and move on to a sense of closure in their relationship with their dying family member.

Processes of Letting Go and Finding Closure for Family Caregivers

- Accept the reality of the diagnosis and prognosis.
- Give up the need to control a situation that cannot be controlled.
- Set boundaries that incorporate self-care strategies to maintain wellness.
- Assist the dying family member in preparation for death.
- Reflect on impending loss and the future without the dying family member.
- Seek information about strategies of caregiving to prevent feelings of inadequacies and incompetence.
- Recognize when to ask for help.

Source: Salmon et al., 2005

Nurses can assist family caregivers by listening and helping them reflect on their understanding of death as an event that cannot be prevented. Nurses can give age and developmentally appropriate information about what occurs as death approaches. They can provide tips and education on caregiving strategies and offer resources that will meet family caregiver needs, such as additional skilled care, support groups, and hospice care.

Closure

In an analysis of the concept of a good death in the literature, Kehl (2006) determined that a sense of closure was an important component of a good death. Closure included finishing unfinished business, preparing for death, and saying goodbye. Family caregivers who are challenged by helping their family member prepare for death also are coping with their future loss and change in their life following the loss (Kwak, Salmon, Acquaviva, Brandt, & Egan, 2007).

The Hospice Experience Model of Care is a framework for explaining what topics and processes can facilitate closure and sense of life completion (Kwak et al., 2007). Based on Byock's (1996) work, the model indicates seven domains of completion and closure:

- life affairs,

- relationships with the community,

- personal relationships,

- experiencing love of self and others,

- accepting finality of life,

- finding meaning, and

- preparing for bereavement.

The Caregiving at Life's End (CGLE) Program, based on this model, helps caregivers develop a sense of life completion and closure in relationships with dying family members. See sidebar for program modules. Learning experiences include facilitated discussion, self-reflection, and self-directed worksheets to guide

conversations between caregivers and care receivers. The curriculum is flexible—
it can be offered for groups or individuals. Most typically, the content is covered
in five sessions, each 1½ hours long, over a few weeks (Kwak et al., 2007). Ideally,
the target audience is those providing care to family members before the final
stages of illness, so there is more time to process their experience and plan for
completion and closure before death is imminent.

Caregiving at Life's End (CGLE) Program Modules

1. The experience of caregiving at the end of life.
2. Aspects of completion and closure for the caregiver and care receiver.
3. Life affairs.
4. Relationships with community.
5. Personal relationships.
6. Experience of love of self and love of others.
7. Acceptance of the finality of life.
8. Meaning of life.
9. Bereavement, renewal, and re-socialization

Source: The Hospice Institute of the Florida Suncoast, 2007

Ending Life and Preparing for Death

Preparation for death results in psychological well-being. People who prepare for
death can take care of legal and financial matters, bring their family and social relationships to closure, and resolve spiritual issues (Chunlestskul, Carlson, Koopmans, & Angen, 2008). As a developmental process, reminiscence to make sense
of one's life (see Chapter 3) helps to achieve what Erikson (1982) called the stage
of ego integrity that leads to a peaceful death. Acknowledging the inevitability of
death and moving away from many of the preoccupations of life allows "authenti-
cally living the rest of one's life" (Chunlestskul et al., p. 6).

Chunlestskul et al. (2008) identified themes of death preparation based on
interviews with women with metastatic breast cancer. The women in the study
viewed working through their death with their family as an opportunity. They

experienced building good memories and helping their family to move on with their own lives after their death. They were able to enjoy daily life. The researchers identified the consequences of death preparation:

- Family and self-growth—the women could help their families as well as themselves;

- Peaceful feelings—they felt free of worrying thoughts and negative emotions and were more ready to face the unknown in death;

- Life lessons—their families learned about death, and they could model acceptance and preparation while enjoying their remaining time with their families.

Chunlestskul et al. (2008) further determined that helping patients to express their feelings about death and to prepare for death is an important interdisciplinary psychosocial intervention. For health care organizations that have a social worker on staff, the social worker may also have an important role in responding to caregiver psychosocial concerns and facilitating a peaceful closure (Baker, 2005).

Themes of Preparation for Death

- *Acknowledging grief*—related to shortened life expectancy, not living to see children and grandchildren grow up, and leaving spouses behind; worried about causing distress to others.

- *Preparing mentally*—through addressing concerns about how to live, changes that need to be made, how to say goodbye, and how families would cope after their death.

- *Seeking information and support*—through individual counseling, group support, printed materials, and other media.

- *Preparing the family*—through talking, professional support, writing, educating others, delegating, and letting go of roles.

- *Preparing for the end of life*—through arranging wills, cleaning out personal effects, arranging for funeral, creating remembrance projects, and living in the present with few regrets.

Source: Chunlestskul, 2008, pp. 8-12

As death becomes imminent, nurses can coach family members in "smoothing the passage" and "nearing death awareness" (Callanan, 1994; Callanan & Kelly, 1992; Perrin, 2006). At life's end, people prepare to detach from life. Their language may be symbolic—about travel or seeing people who have died before them.

Responding to Nearing Death Awareness

- Pay attention to everything a dying person says, because there may be important messages in any communication.

- Help the family listen to the patient's statements and respond with gentle open-ended questions such as, "When does the train leave?" or "Can you tell me what is happening?" or "Can you tell me more?"

- Avoid arguing or challenging the dying person's statements; don't worry about reorienting the patient to present time and place.

- Let the dying person control the conversation, timing, length, and focus.

- Be honest about difficulty understanding. Possible responses include "I think you're trying to tell me something important. I'm trying very hard, but I'm just not getting it. I'll keep trying."

- Show appreciation for the dying person's communication.

- Touch to communicate the message that you are present.

- Remind family members they should continue to communicate verbally with the patient even if unresponsive.

- Families may want to go over some of their favorite memories that show what the dying person meant to them.

- A family member can facilitate letting go by saying, "We will miss you, but we will always love you, and we understand that it is time for you to go."

Sources: Callanan, 1994; Callanan & Kelly, 1992, pp. 241-243; Perrin, 2006, p. 235

Helping Parents Say Goodbye

Accompanying parents on their journey of saying goodbye to a dying child is especially challenging, because parents do not expect their children to die before them. There is a sense of unfairness in having to do such difficult emotional work.

For parents, their dreams and hopes involve their children, and those dreams and hopes are shattered when facing the death of a child. Encourage parents to participate in care and continue in their parental role. Give them permission by asking them what they would like to do for their child or suggesting a specific care activity such as giving a bath. Suggest specific activities that will help to preserve memories—creating a memory box, recording a video, writing letters, and saving a lock of hair or handprints.

Encouraging the family to say goodbye as a group may help to facilitate a sense of support from one another. Ask the family about other supportive resources that would be helpful to them such as spiritual support, friends, or other relatives. Provide privacy if that is what parents want, and give them as much time to say goodbye as they need and is feasible. And, always listen. Units that experience the death of children may want to establish a practice of sending a sympathy card to the parents that acknowledges and gives significance to their very painful loss (Parkman, 1992).

Health Professionals and Saying Goodbye

Nurses also need to consider their own goodbyes to patients. Goodbyes from health professionals convey the value of the relationship and help patients know that they will be remembered (Back, Arnold, Tulsky, Baile, & Fryer-Edwards, 2005). Patients also have the opportunity to say thank you. In an article for physicians about how to say goodbye, the authors suggest many barriers to saying goodbye that are also applicable to nurses:

- fear that saying goodbye communicates they are dying and will make the patient sad,

- uncertainty about prognosis,

- not knowing what to say,

- feeling that it is unprofessional to share emotion, and

- engaging in small talk to avoid facing sadness and loss (Back et al.).

For nurses, who have ongoing care responsibilities, the challenge may be when to say goodbye. The nurse could begin the conversation by saying, "Since neither of us knows exactly how long you have to live, I want to share with you how I have enjoyed knowing you and caring for you." The goodbye becomes a way to express appreciation for the relationship the nurse has experienced with the patient. In addition, provide an opportunity for the patient to respond; acknowledge the patient's emotions; and reaffirm your ongoing commitment to caring for the patient, consistent with your role and responsibilities. Then, after your dialogue with the patient, reflect on your own work and what you have learned from caring for this patient (Back et al., 2005).

Reflective Practice

Working with patients and families to say goodbye involves both an understanding of their needs and an understanding of our own values and beliefs. How would we want to be treated if we were the patient or a family member? What does life completion mean within our own experience?

Reflecting on the personal losses we've experienced can be helpful. For example, an intensive care unit nurse compared the death of one of her patients on a ventilator with the death of her grandmother in hospice. She said, "We knew death was near for Nana, and each of us whispered something important to her. I felt like I truly said goodbye. But for my patient, no one did that because everyone, including myself, was holding out hope that somehow he would make it."

As nurses, we can be present for those patients and family members only when we have a comfort level with the fact that death is natural and inevitable. That presence can falter when we don't care for ourselves and acknowledge our own grief. The pace of the work, especially in busy hospital and skilled nursing facility settings, sometimes makes it difficult to stop and honor the work nurses do with dying patients. If you are feeling the burden of losing patients, advocate for debriefing time and engage other team members. One hospice program begins every team meeting with a ceremony to honor the patients who have died. It is a quiet time to reflect on what those patients and families meant to the staff.

Ethical Practice in Helping Family Members Say Goodbye

ETHICAL PROBLEM: What should I do when a patient is dying and family members are not ready to say goodbye?

What Should I Value?

- Closure for both patient and family members.
- The wishes of patients and family members.
- The knowledge of patients and family members about their family relationships.

Who Should I Be?

- A nurse who facilitates meaningful communication.
- A nurse who respects the needs of both the patient and family members.
- A nurse who offers presence for patients and family members.
- A nurse who is knowledgeable about strategies for assisting patients and families in letting go and finding closure.

What Should I Do?

- Encourage family members to share stories about the patient.
- Encourage family members to arrange their lives so they can be present with the patient as much as possible.
- Ask family members if they would like to be involved in caregiving activities.
- Ask family members what they would like to say to the patient.
- Acknowledge the grieving of family members.
- Ask how family members are coping with the experience.
- Suggest words or phrases to family members that may help their loved one, such as "I love you" and "I will miss you."
- Be present with family members and provide them with the opportunity to reflect on their relationship with the patient.

Nurses' Stories

Cultural Awareness

When working with patients and families, the importance of being aware of different cultural values, norms, and rituals surrounding saying goodbye cannot be overestimated. A hospice nurse relates an experience she had with a Southeast Asian family:

> The family did not want to have their father die in the home. They said that in their tradition, if someone died in a home, the home had to be abandoned because of the bad spirits. When the patient was close to dying, I arranged to have him taken to the hospice unit. The family dressed him carefully and then requested that he be taken through the door feet first. The ambulance attendants were not happy, because it meant making some difficult turns. But I stood my ground because to the patient and family, he was leaving with dignity by going feet first. It was their way of saying goodbye.

Presence

Sometimes our patients die without family or friends. Instead of facilitating the presence and the goodbyes, this hospice nurse provided it:

> The patient was in the nursing home. No friends, no family. He was very near death—having Cheyne-Stokes breathing and periods of apnea. Even though I had a busy day, I sat down beside him and stayed, quietly working on my charting. I had to stop myself from feeling guilty about not rushing off to see other patients. This was my job for the moment and my way of saying good bye to him. I stayed with him for about an hour. He died shortly after I left. I never regretted spending the time.

When family members are with a dying patient, you may need to "walk with them" to encourage them to say goodbye. A Norwegian hospice nurse spoke about a family member who was not ready to say goodbye:

> Right now we have a patient who [receives] artificial intravenous nutrition, and it makes her very sick. She dislikes it, and she tells the nurses and the doctor that she feels she must still do it because of her husband, because he's not prepared, and he needs more time to understand the reality that she's really dying. This is something we are very much aware [of] about the process. It's an art, and we don't always manage, but we try. We are asking questions to make sure they come to some sort of conclusion, and we must just leave it that not all the patients here come to the point where they are ready to give up treatment or ready to say goodbye to their relatives. I think that is the strategy—to walk with them in the process and not to tell them what it should be.

Communicating With Honesty

Patients and families need health professionals to be honest with them. The processes needed for life completion and acceptance of death cannot occur if the information and knowledge are not there. A hospice nurse puts it this way:

> *I think nurses have to learn the gentle skill of being honest with what they are seeing. I think nurses are so hesitant. [Yet] when you see somebody and you've just met them, [it can be important] to find the words [to say], "I'm really concerned because it looks like your mom might not live long."*

Self-Care

To be present for patients and families and to help them in saying goodbye, you need to also acknowledge your own grieving. A hospice nurse talks of journaling as a way to hold onto the meaning of each patient she cares for:

> *A patient I was particularly close to passed. In my sadness and grief, I picked up a paper and began to write. I didn't start at the beginning. I just started a conversation with her. I wrote all the things I missed about seeing her and what she meant to me. Since then I have found great value in writing these stories and re-reading them. When I feel myself caught up in the sadness of patient losses, I sit with these stories—experiencing my connections to the patients all over again.*

Key Points

- Nurses have a significant communication role in guiding and supporting patients with saying goodbye. We can
  - Assist in finding the appropriate words and actions.
  - Facilitate transitions and completion by helping patients and family reflect on the meaning of death, and offer resources to meet those needs.
- Life closure and completion involve accepting the reality of the diagnosis and illness, reflecting on the impending loss and its meaning, setting boundaries for self-care, and seeking help when needed.

- Nurses need to say goodbye to patients and families. This act can be significant in supporting the family as well as maintaining our own well-being.

- Presence is the key to providing the support patients and families need at this time.

REFLECTION QUESTIONS

1. Why is closure at the end of life important to patients and families? What are the benefits?

2. When should a nurse intervene in encouraging the process of saying goodbye for patients and families?

3. What evidence-based strategies for helping patients and family members say goodbye seem most relevant and feasible for you to implement, given your skills, abilities, and personality?

4. How have you been affected by your own experiences of saying goodbye with patients, family members, or friends? What strategies did you use to help you work through saying goodbye and grieving?

References

Back, A. L., Arnold, R. M., Tulsky, J. A., Baile, W. F., & Fryer-Edwards, K. A. (2005). On saying goodbye: Acknowledging the end of the patient-physician relationship with patients who are near death. *Annals of Internal Medicine, 142*(8), 682-686.

Baker, M. (2005). Facilitating forgiveness and peaceful closure: The therapeutic value of psychosocial intervention in end-of-life care. *Journal of Social Work in End-of-Life and Palliative Care, 1*(4), 83-96.

Byock, I. (1996). The nature of suffering and the nature of opportunity at the end of life. *Clinical Geratric Medicine, 12*(2), 237-252.

Byock, I. (2004). *The four things that matter most: A book about living.* New York: Free Press.

Callanan, M. (1994). Farewell messages. *American Journal of Nursing, 94*(5), 19-20.

Callanan, M., & Kelley, P. (1992). *Final gifts: Understanding the special awareness, needs, and communications of the dying.* New York: Bantam Books.

Center on Aging. (2004). *Saying good-bye.* John A. Burns School of Medicine, University of Hawaii. Retrieved August 5, 2008, from www.hawaii.edu/aging

Chunlestskul, K., Carlson, L. E., Koopmans, J. P., & Angen, M. (2008). Lived experiences of Canadian women with metastatic breast cancer in preparation for their death: A qualitative study. *Journal of Palliative Care, 24*(1), 5-15.

Egan, A. K., & Labyak, M. J. (2006). Hospice palliative care: A model for quality end-of-life care. In B. R. Ferrell & N. Coyle (Eds.), *Textbook of palliative nursing* (pp. 13-46). New York: Oxford University Press.

Erikson, E. H. (1982). *The life cycle completed: A review.* New York: Norton.

The Hospice Institute of the Florida Suncoast. (2007). In Kwak , J., Salmon, J. R., Acquaviva, K. D., Brandt, K., & Egan, K. A., Benefits of training family caregivers on experiences of closure during end-of-life care. *Journal of Pain and Symptom Management, 33*(4), 434-445.

Keeley, M. (2007). Turning toward death together: The function of messages during final conversations in close relationships. *Journal of Social and Personal Relationships, 24* (2), 225-253.

Kehl, K. A. (2006). Moving toward peace: An analysis of the concept of a good death. *American Journal of Hospice and Palliative Medicine, 23*(4), 277-286.

Kwak, J., Salmon, J. R., Acquaviva, K. D., Brandt, K., & Egan, K. A. (2007). Benefits of training family caregivers on experiences of closure during end-of-life care. *Journal of Pain and Symptom Management, 33*(4), 434-445.

Lassig, S. L. (2008, Spring). Saying goodbye during a terminal illness. *Family Forum.* Newsletter of the Minnesota Council on Family Relations, pp. 4-5.

Lowrey. S.E. (2008). Communication between the nurse and family caregiver in end-of-life care: A review of literature. *Journal of Hospice and Palliative Nursing, 10(1), 35-45.*

Norlander, L. (2008). *To comfort always: A nurse's guide to end of life care.* Indianapolis, IN: Sigma Theta Tau International.

Parkman, S. E. (1992). Helping families say good-bye. *The American Journal of Maternal Child Nursing, 17,* 14-17.

Perrin, K. (2006). Communicating with seriously ill and dying patients, their families, and their health care providers. In M. L. Matzo & D. W. Sherman (Eds.), *Palliative care nursing: Quality care to the end of life* (pp. 221-245). New York: Springer.

Poor, B., & Gary, E. (2001). Communicating with the dying patient. In B. Poor & G. P. Poirrier, (Eds.), *End of life nursing care* (pp. 213-226). Sudbury, MA: Jones and Bartlett.

Prince-Paul, M. (2008). Understanding the meaning of social well-being at end of life. *Oncology Nursing Forum, 35*(3). 365-371.

Salmon, J. R., Kwak, J., Acquavia, K. D., Brandt, B., & Egan, K. A. (2005). Transformative aspects of caregiving at life's end. *Journal of Pain and Symptom Management, 29*(2), 121-129.

Swigart, V., Lidz, C., Butterworth, V., & Arnold, R. (1996). Letting go: Family willingness to forgo life support. *Heart & Lung, 26*(6), 483-494.

*A Native American elder was talking about his culture
to a group of hospice nurses. We kept asking him specific
questions like, "Will I offend if I use the word 'dying'?"
I remember how patiently he tried to answer all the
questions, but a lot of his answers were, "I don't know."
Finally he said, "We're all different, just like you are. The
best way to find the answer for each person is to ask."*

—Hospice nurse

8

•

Responding to Cultural Needs in End-of-Life Care

Culture is a part of all our communication—verbal and nonverbal. We bring our own culture and beliefs into interactions with patients and families. They, in turn, bring their own cultural background and experiences. Our medical model can conflict with the values and beliefs of our patients. We need to be especially aware of how our beliefs, the beliefs of our patients, and the culture of our health care system play a significant role in communication at the end of life.

Meaning of Culture

Culture refers to the knowledge, values, beliefs, and habits of a population or society that can be differentiated from other societal groups (Lewis, Heitkemper, & Dirksen, 2004). Leininger (2002) emphasizes that beliefs, values, and life patterns of a cultural group are shared, transmitted to subsequent generations, and influence how people think and approach life. Helman (1994) adds that culture provides guidelines about how to see the world, how to relate to others and the natural environment, and how to act. Hallenbeck (2001) explains that culture is much more than ethnicity; many factors combine to create cultural identity—"race; national origin; religion; age; gender; sexual orientation; and family, professional, and community roles" (p. 402). An important component of developing cultural identity is socialization into the culture that results over time through the imprinting of societal structures—religious, social system, and artistic and intellectual experiences within the culture (Giger, Davidhizar, & Fordham, 2006). The meaning given to illness, suffering, and death develops out of these cultural experiences (Kagawa-Singer & Blackhall, 2001).

Universal Needs in End-of-Life Care

Although there are variations in communication about end-of-life choices and decision-making and responses to dying based on culture, there are also many themes that apply to all cultural groups, based on a common humanity.

Duffy and colleagues conducted 10 focus groups, stratified by race and gender, with 73 participants (Duffy, Jackson, Schim, Ronis, & Fowler, 2006a; 2006b). In discussion of common end-of-life scenarios, end-of-life concepts identified as important by all cultural groups were

- being comfortable,
- experiencing good communication with the physician,
- having someone take care of their perceived responsibilities,
- having hope and optimism, and
- having their spiritual beliefs honored.

Dying with dignity is also a desire of persons in all cultures (Kemp, 2005). Other end-of-life concepts that most cultural groups identified as important in the study by Duffy et al. were

- experiencing love and compassion;
- having care needs met;

- having the opportunity to express feelings;

- fixing relationships, if needed;

- saying goodbye;

- having choices;

- making plans;

- avoiding pain; and

- being "ready to go."

Cultural Variations Related to End-of-Life Care

Although there are variations in preferences for communication and end-of-life care across cultures, we must treat each person as an individual. Because of life experience and acculturation, any one person may have preferences different from what we have come to know through research and interactions with a cultural group.

African-American Perspectives

In the focus groups conducted by Duffy et al. (2006a; 2006b), Black participants expressed a preference for having end-of-life care in an intensive care unit, hospice, or nursing home rather than being at home. They did not want to be a burden to family members. However, in a review of research, Doolen and York (2007) suggest that Blacks believe that the voice of the family is more important than a written document such as an advance directive (AD). Proportionately, they are much less likely to use hospice services and palliative care services (Hopp & Duffy, 2000). Because African Americans distrust the U.S. health care system, which has historically provided them less access to health care in comparison to the White population, they are likely to regard advance directive planning and withholding aggressive treatment with suspicion (Hallenbeck, 2001; West & Levi, 2004). African Americans want family members involved in their care (Barclay, Blackhall, & Tulsky, 2007; Sherman, 2006). As a result, they may see less of a need for ADs. They may also be less likely to ask for pain and symptom management because of an expectation that they must endure suffering (West & Levi, 2004). In the study by Duffy and colleagues, African-American women preferred that everything should be done to maintain life, because the physician might have made a mistake in predicting prognosis, while African-American men wanted all treatment except for life support (Duffy et al., 2006a; 2006b).

Hispanic Perspectives

Hispanics view life as a gift from God, see death as natural, and do not want to be a burden to their families (Mitty, 2001). In the focus groups conducted by Duffy and colleagues (2006a; 2006b), Hispanic-Latino participants wanted to avoid nursing homes but were open to hospitals and hospice services for end-of-life care. However, most participants were unfamiliar with hospice (Sullivan, 2001). One-third of participants did not want disclosure about their illness, believing that knowing about their terminal illness might increase illness and the likelihood of dying.

Like African Americans, Hispanics believe that the family is the most important decision maker, in comparison to use of ADs, and were less likely to use specific health care proxies as well as ADs (Barclay et al., 2007; Doolen & York, 2007; Jenko & Moffit, 2006; Sherman, 2006; Valente, 2004). Hispanics are more often focused on the present, which can lead to a disinterest in advance planning (Mitty, 2001). Duffy and colleagues found a major gender difference in Hispanic views about medical intervention at the end of life. Hispanic women were more likely to want more aggressive intervention in comparison to Hispanic men, who said they would refuse interventions such as dialysis and pain medication so they could stay alert (Duffy et al., 2006a; 2006b).

Asian and Pacific Islander Perspectives

Research on views about end-of-life treatment and care has been explored for many Asian cultures, including Korean American, Japanese, and Hmong. Generally, depending on the level of acculturation, Asians are more likely to emphasize decision making in the context of what is best for the family. Elderly family members are revered and protected, and family members may not want them involved in decision-making so that their final days will be peaceful.

It may be difficult to assess the needs of Asian patients who respect authority and are reluctant to complain about their discomfort (Sherman, 2006). Asian families may also refuse hospice services, because they are obligated to care for their dying relative. For some Asian families, their duty to care for dying family members may mean they wish to have aggressive measures to preserve life (Searight & Gafford, 2005). Use of ADs is also lower in Asian populations in comparison to Caucasians in the United States (Jenko & Moffitt, 2006), although rates of having an AD and health care proxy are higher in comparison to other minority groups (Valente, 2004).

In Asian cultures outside the U.S., directly informing a patient of a cancer diagnosis is considered to be cruel; in Japan, physicians often use terms that are more indirect when discussing cancer (Searight & Gafford, 2005). Withholding truth about a diagnosis of terminal illness is consistent with Japanese culture. It means doing good for the patient, since disclosure about bad news could result in a patient giving up and dying or becoming depressed and committing suicide, based on Japanese perspectives (Davis & Konishi, 2000).

Hmong Americans also emphasize family interdependence in decision-making about end of life (Gerdner, Cha, Yang, & Tripp-Reimer, 2007). The family group is responsible for decision-making under the guidance of the eldest male. It is considered bad luck to discuss or make plans for death, because that may cause premature death. Certain phrases may be acceptable, such as "last breath" and "reaching the 120th year of life," which is consistent with a Hmong folk tale about the ideal age for the end of life. Death at home may be preferred to provide rest for the spirit. Hmong may view the hospice philosophy of not offering life-prolonging interventions as disrespectful.

Native American Perspectives

Similar to Hispanics, Native Americans think of life and death as a natural process (Sherman, 2006). The Navajo expect people to speak positively to one another, because they believe language and thought influences what happens (Mitty, 2001). This means that truth telling, as in giving bad news about expected end-of-life outcomes, is taboo. Discussions of ADs and support that will be needed may not be discussed in the Navajo culture, because the discussions are considered harmful (Searight & Gafford, 2005).

Arab American Perspectives

Arab Americans want to be informed about their prognosis, so they can make peace on earth in order to get into heaven. In studies by Duffy et al. (2006a, 2006b), Arab American participants did not want aggressive or heroic treatment and did not want to be in a nursing home. Family members were expected to care for dying relatives, and they were unfamiliar with the availability of hospice. Arab Americans who are Muslims are more comfortable interacting with health care staff of the same gender (Kemp, 2005).

European American Perspective

In contrast to other cultures, European Americans generally do not think it is their family's responsibility to care for them at the end of life (Duffy et al., 2006a; 2006b). Typically, they want to know what to expect, have choices, avoid pain and heroic measures, and have greater interest in completing an AD and identifying a health care proxy (Hopp & Duffy, 2000). Independence, autonomy, and individual control in end-of-life decision-making are valued by many people in this group (Valente, 2004). European Americans are the most negative about life support and are less likely to want their lives prolonged through technological advances (Blackhall et al., 1999).

Gender Perspectives

Some difference between genders exists in certain cultures concerning attitudes toward the use of life support. This difference may lead to a decision that is not consistent with a patient's wishes, given that spouses often make decisions regarding treatment at the end of life (Duffy et al., 2006a; 2006b). One gender difference that Duffy and colleagues noted in focus group responses indicated that, in comparison to men, women more often wanted touch, prayer, mental awareness, and resolution of unfinished business at the end of life.

The Culture of the Health Care System and Health Professionals

Health care in the United States is shaped by values that indicate the sacredness of life, autonomous decision-making, and avoiding needless suffering (Kagawa-Singer, 1998). This means that the idea of withholding the opportunity for informed consent is not compatible with mainstream health care practices (Giger, Davidhizar, & Fordham, 2006). Nurses who promote truth telling, informed consent, and ADs with all their patients and families, consistent with the value of autonomy in the U.S. health care system, will in some situations be culturally insensitive and ignore their patient's needs and views (Solomon, 1999). Solomon suggests that autonomy should be offered as an invitation, but not as a command or assumption. For some cultures, promoting good and preventing harm through providing information is more important than autonomy (Searight & Gafford, 2005). Efforts to control end-of-life experiences may seem wrong and unnatural to those whose culture guides them to view death as natural and part of the life cycle (Sherman, 2006). For nurses, the cultural values of the health care system and the nursing profession, developed through education and socialization into the profession, as well as their own cultural background influence responses to dying patients and their families (Mazanec & Panke, 2006).

Cultural Norms for End-of-Life Issues

Communication patterns are determined by cultural norms. Nurses who understand the variations in cultural norms will be more effective in meeting the needs of their patients and families in end-of-life care.

Truth Telling and Disclosure

Structures and processes in the U.S. health care system support the provision of direct, honest, clear, and timely health information. This approach is in contrast with cultural beliefs that family members should protect their dying family member from harmful information that takes away their hope (Turner, 2002). Health care professionals may feel "caught in the middle" as they attempt to honor the informed consent process while being sensitive to family "wants" about nondisclosure of bad news. Searight and Gafford (2005) summarized four primary reasons for nondisclosure of bad news, from other cultural perspectives:

- People from certain cultures specifically view discussion of serious illness as disrespectful or impolite.

- Some believe that open discussion of serious illness may provoke unnecessary depression or anxiety in the patient.

- Some believe that direct disclosure may eliminate hope.

- Some believe that speaking aloud about a condition, even in a hypothetical sense, makes death or terminal illness real because of the power of the spoken word (p. 517).

Touch

Touch can effectively communicate caring and support to dying patients and their families; however, there is great variation among cultures in comfort with touch. Although it is a norm for health care professionals to touch others through many caregiving procedures, deliberate touch apart from physical caregiving may be experienced differently than intended. Typically, cultures in which individuals hold their emotions close may be uncomfortable with public touch. These include English, German, Scandinavian, and Chinese cultures. Cultures that seem to be comfortable with touch and welcome it include Latino, Middle Eastern, and Jewish cultures (Poor & Gary, 2001).

Advance Directives and Health Care Proxy

The formalized and legalized process of ADs in the U.S. is based on the 1991 Patient Self-Determination Act (PSDA). The values that resulted in passage of the PSDA are the same as those that drive health care practices: patient autonomy, informed decision-making, truth telling, and patient control over the dying process (Giger et al., 2006). From the above discussion of different cultural perspectives, it is apparent that the act of completing an AD and identifying a health care proxy is not consistent with the values of many cultures. For patients and families who are present-oriented, wish to leave what will happen to God, are oriented to family versus individual decision-making, or mistrust the motives of a health care system—an emphasis on AD completion may be met with resistance or confusion (Turner, 2002).

Cultural Competence

Cultural competence begins with appreciating the differences among ethnic groups and wanting to improve relationships across cultures (Bigby, 2003; Hallenbeck & Goldstein, 1999). Reflection and critique of your attitudes and responses to difference are important for developing cultural competence. Jenko and Moffit (2006) developed a self-discovery questionnaire that includes questions about (a) negative and positive perceptions about a person's racial-ethnic identity; (b) socialization experiences that influence values and responses of other cultures, including historical experience of encountering someone with a terminal illness; (c) encounters with differences, such as disability, abuse of drugs, and imprisonment; (d) exploration of values about food and time; and (e) cultural characteristics that seem difficult to understand.

McPhatter (1997) developed a cultural competence attainment model that begins with knowledge development, moves to changing a person's views, and finally results in building skill in cross-cultural interactions (Reese, Melton, & Ciaravino, 2004). More specifically, the model includes the following three components:

- **A grounded knowledge base** that involves analysis and reformulation by including knowledge generated by communities of color, both traditional and nontraditional institutions, and other professional disciplines.

- **An enlightened consciousness** that results from a revised worldview.

- **Cumulative skill proficiency,** which is ongoing and involves valuing the worldviews of others, engaging in interactions with culturally diverse individuals and groups, and developing cross-cultural communication skills.

A cultural competence model developed by Schim and Miller (Doorenbos & Schim, 2004) has four components of cultural competence:

1. **Cultural diversity** involves recognition of the unique values, beliefs, and customs of diverse populations in a society.

2. **Cultural awareness** involves exchanging information about cultural variations.

3. **Cultural sensitivity** involves development of effective communication skills—listening, touching, use of space, language patterns, and use of translators.

4. **Cultural competence** involves use of the above behaviors daily in nursing practice.

In culturally competent end-of-life care, nurses provide interventions that take into account the cultural meaning of a good death; incorporate cultural food traditions into care; and are consistent with cultural traditions of including family in end-of-life care, as well as care of the body following death. In addition, cultural competence involves "individualization," which means that nurses assess individual needs so that they do not stereotype or assume needs based only on a person's cultural background.

Cultural Assessment

The End-of-Life Nursing Education Consortium (ELNEC) suggests using the CONFHER model for a brief cultural assessment (Fong, 1985; City of Hope National Medical Center and the American Association of Colleges of Nursing, 2003). The CONFHER Model organizes assessment questions into seven categories:

1. **C**ommunication—primary language, use of health terms, and nonverbal communication.

2. **O**rientation—ethnic identity and place of birth.

3. **N**utrition—food preferences and taboos.

4. Family relationships—family structure and decision-making, head of household, and role of women.

5. Health and health beliefs—explanation of illness and measures to stay healthy.

6. Education—learning style, educational level, and occupation.

7. Religion—religious beliefs or restrictions that affect health or illness.

Zerwekh (2006) suggests assessing type of greeting, personal space needed, use of eye contact, comfort with touch, and conversational style. The Giger-Davidhizar transcultural model has been specifically applied to assist health professionals in assessing end-of-life concerns and decision-making (Giger et al., 2006). Assessment questions address communication patterns, space needs in terms of closeness, time orientation, beliefs about control over self and environment, social relationships in family and religious systems, and variations in expression of pain. Communication assessment questions specifically explore family decision-making, trust in relationships, and patterns of expression.

Nursing Interventions

Developing Awareness

Based on models of cultural competence, developing awareness involves acquiring knowledge about cultural variations and similarities and also reflecting on how your own cultural beliefs influence nursing care. By looking into the available evidence on culture and end-of-life care, nurses can incorporate their learning about the beliefs, customs, and values of patients and families from various cultures into their end-of-life care (Doolen & York, 2007). Strategies for increasing cultural awareness include

* Health professional education, focus groups with patients, programs developed to respond to care recommendations for specific cultural groups.

- Examining beliefs and biases (Barclay et al., 2007).

- Speaking with someone who represents a specific culture about cultural meanings of end of life and possible taboos (Sherman, 2006).

- Learning about features of nonverbal communication that are culturally appropriate, such as use of gestures, eye contact, touch, and space preferred for face-to-face interactions (Mazanec & Panke, 2006).

"When interacting with patients and their families, learning about what a good death means to them is important, rather than assuming the meaning of a good death based on your own beliefs."

Relationships

Focusing on relationship development can greatly improve intercultural communication. When interacting with patients and their families, learning about what a good death means to them is important, rather than assuming the meaning of a good death based on your own beliefs (West & Levi, 2004). Work to build trusting relationships through giving time for discussion and following up on that discussion (Raghaven, Smith, & Arnold, 2008). Consider different worldviews when working to develop goals that are mutually determined (Giger et al., 2006). Respect for difference and cultural background is essential to working through mutual goal setting (Hallenbeck & Goldstein, 1999).

Use of Translators-Interpreters

When translators or interpreters are needed, it is important to note that complete accuracy is difficult to achieve. Using family members as interpreters should be avoided, because they may have great difficulty communicating bad news, may misinterpret news, and sometimes avoid topics related to body functions (Kemp, 2005; Barclay et al., 2007).

Facilitating Decision-Making

Show respect for cultural norms on preferences for disclosure by giving an option to refuse disclosure (Searight & Gafford, 2005). View the family as the unit for autonomy in situations where the cultural norm is family decision-making. Frame the situation as one in which the family takes responsibility for making choices that show consideration of what is good for the entire family (Barclay et al., 2007). Work with the interdisciplinary health care team to offer patients the opportunity to make their own end-of-life decision or delegate decisions to family members (Blackhall et al., 1999). Offer opportunities for continued dialogue, because openness and need to talk can vary with changes in the patient's condition and outlook. Remember, the choices of any one individual are not determined solely by the ethnic group (Hallenbeck & Goldstein, 1999).

Questions for Exploration of Preferences for Disclosure and Decision-Making

- How much do you want to know? (Mitty, 2001, p. 31)
- Who besides yourself do you want informed? (Mitty, 2001, p. 31)
- Who do you want to be with you when treatment outcomes are discussed? (Mitty, 2001, p. 31)
- Some people want to know everything about their medical condition, and others do not. What is your preference? (Jenko & Moffit, 2006, p. 179)
- Do you prefer to make medical decisions about tests and treatments for yourself, or would you prefer that someone else make them for you? (Jenko & Moffit, 2006, p. 179)
- What do you want to know about your condition? (Lapine et al., 2001, p. 478)
- Whom do you want to know about your condition? (Lapine et al., 2001, p. 478)
- Whom should we talk to about your treatments and potential outcomes? (Lapine et al., 2001, p. 478)
- Whom do you want to make health care decisions for you? (Lapine et al., 2001, p. 478)

Educational Strategies

Although some ethnic groups may be reluctant to use hospice services, education about what is offered may increase their receptiveness. Family members can benefit from education about how they can contribute to decision-making at the end of life. One example is educational booklets that were designed for family caregivers in Honolulu, Hawaii, to improve their knowledge and practices related to end-of-life decision-making and caregiving issues (Braun, Karel, & Zir, 2006). The population included Asians, Whites, and Pacific Islanders. An evaluation through pre-tests and post-tests of 570 participants showed that receptivity to hospice increased for all participant groups, and there were increases in number of living wills for elders and in both caregivers and elders who had funeral or burial plans. However, Pacific Islanders knew the least about advance directives, both pre- and post-test, and their AD completion rate was significantly lower than for the other groups. The authors suggested that planning for end of life might not be important for Pacific Islanders, who experience more poverty and a lower life expectancy. Go to the Web site at www.hawaii.edu/aging to download the educational booklet.

Reflective Practice

The best way to gain perspective on cultural practices, values, and beliefs regarding communication at the end of life is to step out of our "cultural shoes." A White hospice nurse best described the "aha" moment when she was talking with an African-American family about the benefits of hospice: "I believe so strongly that hospice is the best care for dying patients and that the hospice benefits are the best the health care system can provide. I was shocked when one of the family members turned to me and said, 'Why are you trying to give us all these things? Don't you think we can take care of our own?'" Later, the nurse reflected on the conversation. "I imagined myself in their place. What if someone from the African American community came to my home and said, 'Trust us, we know how to take care of your dying loved one.' I realized my own arrogance and ignorance in presenting to them that I knew what was best."

As we walk with our patients and families through this difficult journey, it is important to stop, listen, and recognize that our knowledge and beliefs might not be the same as theirs. This is a time to be present and listen. It is also a time to ask rather than tell.

We need to discern our own values and recognize that although promoting good and preventing harm are foundational to nursing, when it comes to end-of-life care options and decision-making, autonomy is really a primary value for most health care professionals. However, we cannot assume that autonomy motivates all our patients in expressing their preferences.

Ethical Practice in Cultural Awareness Regarding Disclosure

ETHICAL PROBLEM: What should I do when a daughter does not want her mother to know she is dying, when I believe the patient has a right to know so that she can prepare for death?

What Should I Value?

* What it means to you to provide good end-of-life care.

* The cultural values of the daughter and mother about disclosure of bad news.

* Nursing knowledge about what it means to provide culturally competent care.

Who Should I Be?

* A nurse who respects the uniqueness of each patient and family and the cultural background they bring to the health care environment.

* A nurse who recognizes different viewpoints about preferences for knowing about prognosis and expected outcomes.

* A nurse who is willing to advocate for the family decision-making model.

What Should I Do?

* Convene an interdisciplinary team meeting to discuss cultural aspects that are motivating family preferences, and develop consensus on strategies that support family preferences.

- Explain the informed consent process to the daughter, and that it is a custom of the health care organization.

- Discuss with the daughter possible benefits of the mother knowing more about her prognosis (concerning preparation for death), as well as the daughter's concerns about potential negative outcomes of disclosure.

- Defer to the daughter's decision about what is best for her mother.

Systems, by their nature, try to make things the same for streamlining, convenience, and cost-effectiveness. The challenge is to create a system that allows for or even embraces difference. If we are truly being culturally competent, we need to look beyond our individual interactions with patients and families to examine systems of care. Can we create a culturally competent system that does not require patients to negotiate to receive recognition of the cultural aspects of their health care? I think we need to use words such as working together and collaborating in place of negotiating as we work toward developing cultural competence.

An important virtue in this endeavor is humility—we have a lot to learn about best strategies for culturally competent care. All nurses who are involved in any aspect of end-of-life care can work to develop a more culturally competent workforce. Administrators can provide time, space, and funds for cross-cultural education; create opportunities for debriefing about end-of-life care for culturally diverse patients and families; discuss needed system changes; and evaluate cultural competence in patient care and systems. Educators can integrate cultural aspects into their work in a variety of educational formats. Nurses on the front line of patient and family end-of-life care can seek and apply evidence about best practices for culturally competent care and can raise questions with colleagues about how to best meet cultural needs in working with patients and families.

Nurses' Stories

Decision-making

Our health care culture values patient autonomy and decision-making. If a patient is unable to make a decision, the proxy—often the next of kin, such as a spouse—must step in. In some cultures, the decision makers might be someone else, as in the following example.

> I had this patient, a man in his 40s with a brain tumor who was from the Middle East. He lived with his wife. Part of what we do when we admit a patient is to talk about comfort care and treatment decisions. The patient was too sick and too confused to talk. When I asked the wife about resuscitation and hospitalization preferences, she shook her head. "I can't say. I can't make that decision." We had to wait for the brother who lived in another state to come before we could proceed with hospice care. The brother wanted him to be hospitalized and treated. Even though I thought it was adding to his suffering, I had to respect the decision.

Communication and Use of Interpreters

Often one of the greatest challenges for nurses is communicating with a patient and family who do not speak English. Even when using trained language interpreters, it is important to consider that the interpreter also comes with his or her own background, experience, values, and beliefs. A hospice nurse talks about her experience using an interpreter during a home visit with a dying patient.

> I was so busy trying to deal with the patient's symptoms and trying to get his breathing more relaxed that I didn't pay much attention to the interpreter. It was a long visit and by the time we left the house, I could see that the interpreter was exhausted. We stopped on the front sidewalk, and I thanked her for her work. She looked at me and said, "That was the hardest thing I've ever done. I've never talked with anyone about dying before." I realized that the interpreter was part of the care team, and I hadn't prepared her for what was happening. Next time, before I go into a home with an interpreter, I'm going to talk with her or him about what to expect. I mean, really, we do that with all our other team members; we should do it with the interpreters.

Respecting Values and Beliefs

The beliefs, rituals, and values of our patients might not be the same as ours. However, an important aspect of communicating at the end of life is demonstrating acceptance and respect for others. An ICU nurse tells of how she worked with a family and physician to create mutual respect:

> I had this African American family who wanted the doctor to pray with them. I knew he was Jewish, but I told him that it was important to the family to be with them. He stayed with them. It was amazing–it only took a little advocating on my part.

A Norwegian hospice nurse struggled with being consistent with both the hospice philosophy and cultural values in talking about death in Norway.

> In [our] culture we don't talk a lot about death. It's taboo in our culture as well as in many other Western civilizations. We're so far away from dying. A son did not want to talk about the end of life of his mother. He did not want her to come to hospice. He said, "I don't want her to come because she's not going to die, and if she comes, you cannot talk to her about death." That's a cultural barrier we meet sometimes.

Key Points

- Patients from all cultures and backgrounds have common needs at the end of life. These include
    - comfort.
    - communication,
    - having care needs met.
    - respect for cultural beliefs,
    - fixing relationships, and
    - saying goodbye.

- Preferences for communication at the end of life vary from culture to culture, as do preferences for treatment and care.

- Western health care practice is based on the concepts of autonomy and informed consent and can be in conflict with cultural beliefs.

- Cultural competence includes a nurse's self-awareness and appreciation for variations among the patients and families cared for.

REFLECTION QUESTIONS

1. What are your cultural values about dying and end-of-life care?

2. How do mainstream health care system values influence end-of-life care strategies and communication?

3. What communication strategies can you use in situations in which cultural differences challenge your usual approaches to end-of-life care?

References

Barclay, J. S., Blackhall, L. J., & Tulsky, J. A. (2007). Communication strategies in cultural issues in the delivery of bad news. *Journal of Palliative Medicine, 10*(4), 958-977.

Bigby, J. (2003). Beyond culture: Strategies for caring for patients from diverse racial, ethnic, and cultural groups. In J. Bigby (Ed.), *Cross-cultural medicine* (pp. 1-28). Philadelphia: American College of Physicians.

Blackhall, L. J., Frank, G., Murphy, S. T., Michel, V., Palmer, J. M., & Azen, S. P. (1999). Ethnicity and attitudes towards life sustaining technology. *Social Science & Medicine, 48*, 1779-1789.

Braun, K. L., Karel, H., & Zir, A. (2006). Family response to end-of-life education: Differences by ethnicity and stage of caregiving. *American Journal of Hospice & Palliative Medicine, 23*(4), 269-276.

City of Hope National Medical Center and the American Association of Colleges of Nursing. (2003). *End-of-Life Nursing Education Consortium (ELNEC) Graduate Curriculum.*

Davis, A. J., & Konishi, E. (2000). End-of-life ethical issues in Japan. *Geriatric Nursing, 21*(2), 89-91.

Doolen, J., & York, N. L. (2007). Cultural differences with end-of-life care in the critical care unit. *Dimensions of Critical Care Nursing, 26*(5), 194-198.

Doorenbos, A. & Schim, S. (2004). Cultural competence in hospice. *American Journal of Hospice and Palliative Care, 21*(1), 28-32.

Duffy, S. A., Jackson, F. C., Schim, S. M., Ronis, D. L., & Fowler, K. E. (2006a). Cultural concepts at the end of life. *Nursing Older People, 18*(8), 10-14.

Duffy, S. A., Jackson, F. C., Schim, S. M., Ronis, D. L., & Fowler, K. E. (2006b). Racial/ethnic preferences, sex preferences, and perceived discrimination related to end-of-life care. *Journal of the American Geriatrics Society, 54*(1), 150-157.

Fong, C. M. (1985). Ethnicity in nursing practice. *Topics in Clinical Nursing, 7*(3), 1-10.

Gerdner, L. A., Cha, D., Yang, D., & Tripp-Reimer, T. (2007). The circle of life: End-of-life care and death rituals for Hmong-American elders. *Journal of Geronotological Nursing, 33*(5), 20-29.

Giger, J. N., Davidhizar, R. E., & Fordham, P. (2006). Multi-cultural and multi-ethnic considerations and advanced directives: Developing cultural competency. *Journal of Cultural Diversity, 13*(1), 3-9.

Hallenbeck, J. L. (2001). Intercultural differences and communication at the end of life. *Primary Care, 28*(2), 401-413.

Hallenbeck, J., & Goldstein, M. K. (1999). Cultural considerations beyond medical ethics. *Generations, 23*(1), 24-29.

Helman, C. G. (1994). *Culture health and illness.* London: Butterworth Heinemann.

Hopp, F. P., & Duffy, S. A. (2000). Racial variations in end-of-life care. *Journal of the American Geriatrics Society, 48*(6), 658-663.

Jenko, M., & Moffitt, S. R. (2006). Transcultural nursing principles: An application to hospice care. *Journal of Hospice and Palliative Nursing, 8*(3), 172-180.

Kagawa-Singer, M. (1998). The cultural context of death rituals and mourning practices. *Oncology Nursing Forum, 25*(1), 1725-1756.

Kagawa-Singer, M. & Blackhall, L. (2001). Negotiating cross-cultural issues at the end of life. *JAM A, 286,* 2993-3001.

Kemp, C. (2005). Cultural issues in palliative care. *Seminars in Oncology Nursing, 21*(1), 44-52.

Lapine, A., Wang-Cheng, R., Goldstein, M., Nooney, A., Lamb, G., & Derse, A. R. (2001). When cultures clash: Physician, patient, and family wishes in truth disclosure for dying patients. *Journal of Palliative Medicine, 4*(4), 475-480.

Leininger, M. (2002). Transcultural nursing and globalization of health care: Importance, focus, and historical aspects. In M. Leininger & M. R. McFarland (Eds.), *Transcultural nursing* (pp. 3-43). New York: McGraw-Hill.

Lewis, S. M., Heitkemper, M. M., & Dirksen, S. T. (2004*). Medical surgical nursing: Assessment and management of clinical problems.* St. Louis, MO: Mosby.

Mazanec, P., & Panke, J. T. Cultural considerations in palliative care. (2006). In B. R. Ferrell & N. Coyle (Eds.). *Textbook of palliative nursing* (pp. 623-633). New York: Oxford University Press.

McPhatter, A. R. (1997). Cultural competence in child welfare: What is it? How do we achieve it? What happens without it? *Child Welfare, 76*, 255-278.

Mitty, E. L. (2001). Removing cultural blinders. *Reflections on Nursing Leadership, 27*(1), 29-46.

Poor, B., & Gary, E. (2001). Communicating with the dying patient. In B. Poor & G. P. Poirrier (Eds.), *End of life nursing care* (pp. 213-226). Sudbury, MA: Jones and Bartlett.

Raghavan, M., Smith, A., & Arnold, R. (2008). Fast fact and concept #204: African Americans and end-of-life care. End-of-Life/Palliative Education Resource Center. Retrieved April 17, 2009, from http://www.eperc.mcw.edu

Reese, D. J., Melton, E., & Ciaravino, K. (2004). Programmatic barriers to providing culturally competent end-of-life care. *American Journal of Hospice & Palliative Medicine, 21*(5), 357-364.

Searight, H. R., & Gafford, J. (2005). Cultural diversity at the end of life: Issues and guidelines for family physicians. *American Family Physician, 71*(3), 515-522.

Sherman, D. W. (2006). Spirituality and culture as domains of quality palliative care. In M. L. Matzo & D. W. Sherman (Eds.), *Palliative Care Nursing: Quality care to the end of life* (pp. 3-49). New York: Springer.

Solomon, M. Z. (1999). Why are advance directives a non-issue outside the United States? *Innovations in End-of-life care, 1*(1). Retrieved April 17, 2009, from http://www2.edc.org/last-acts/archivesJan99/default.asp.

Sullivan, M. C. (2001). Lost in translation: How Latinos view end-of-life care. *Plastic Surgical Nursing, 21*(2), 90-91.

Turner, L. (2002). Bioethics and end-of-life care in multi-ethnic settings: Cultural diversity in Canada and the USA. *Mortality, 7*(3), 285-301.

Valente, S. M. (2004). End of life and ethnicity. *Journal for Nurses in Staff Development, 29*(6), 285-293.

West, S. K. & Levi, L. (2004). Culturally appropriate end-of-life care for the black American. *Home Healthcare Nurse, 22*(3), 164-168.

Zerwekh, J. V. (2006). *Nursing care at the end of life.* Philadelphia: F. A. Davis.

I sat through a family conference with a wonderful doctor. The patient was in a coma, and they were talking about a feeding tube. The doctor read from the patient's directive that said no feeding tube. He said, "You are so fortunate that your mother made these decisions for you." Then he went around the room and checked with everyone to make sure they understood and were in agreement. Every single one of them said, "Mom wouldn't want that (the feeding tube)."

–Hospital nurse

9

•

Advance Care Planning

A century ago, most people died of acute illnesses. Few treatment options existed that could either save or prolong life. Today, most people die from chronic illnesses and conditions with many different possible treatments and choices along the way. Patients are often walking a fine line between treatments that can prolong living and treatments that can prolong dying. Nurses have an important role to play in facilitating the discussion and providing the information that can help patients and families make choices during this difficult journey.

Advance Care Planning

Advance care planning (ACP) is a thoughtful, facilitated discussion about care wishes and goals at the end of life. It encompasses a lifetime of values and beliefs and is not simply a discussion of medical treatment choices (Norlander & McSteen, 2000). As a concept, ACP is broader than advance directives (AD). An AD may be the outcome of advance care planning. The goal of ACP is to develop a shared understanding of a patient's values and preferences for end-of-life health care decisions (Moore, 2005). ACP supports patient autonomy by providing an opportunity for decision-making while a patient has decisional capacity. Components of ACP include

- Determination of care and treatment goals, including values.
- Possible initiation and completion of an AD.
- Decision-making about specific treatment options (CPR and life-sustaining treatment such as ventilation, feeding tubes, and dialysis).
- Involvement of family and other social system support (Dahlin & Giansiracusa, 2006; Moore, 2005).

ACP is a social process that has benefits for relationships, because discussion with family members can clarify what patients want, relieve the burden of decision-making for family members, and reduce the potential for family conflict by avoiding decision-making in an emergency situation (Dahlin & Giansiracusa, 2006; Pearlman, Cole, Patrick, Starks, & Cain, 1995). ACP discussions will be most effective if they take place over time to allow patients opportunity for reflection and for involvement of family and friends (Dahlin & Giansiracusa).

Advance Directives

Advance directives are legal, written documents outlining treatment wishes at the end of life when patients can no longer speak for themselves. The United States Congress passed the Patient Self Determination Act (PSDA) in 1990 to encourage autonomous end-of-life decision-making by requiring that all health care providers who receive Medicare and Medicaid funds provide written information about the existence of or the opportunity for advance directives (Soskis, 1997). To facilitate advance care planning, nurses need to be familiar with the legal form of advance directives specific to their state and the concepts of advance care planning. Three purposes for advance directives identified by Matzo and Ramsey (2006) include:

1. ADs give people the opportunity to direct the kind of health care they want, should they not have the ability to make their own decisions in the future.

2. ADs provide direction to health care professionals for decisions on the use of life-sustaining treatment in situations where patients lack decision-making capacity.

3. ADs protect health care providers and organizations from civil and criminal liability.

Benefits of ADs include an emphasis on quality of life, reduction of burden of decision-making for family members, preservation of dignity in health care, control over life decisions, and preservation of life savings (Valente, 2004). ADs can also prevent future conflict when people become cognitively impaired (Duke & Thompson, 2007.) Content of advance directives should include:

1. Descriptions of health care treatments that are wanted or not wanted.

2. Instructions for when the directive should be initiated.

3. Identification of the surrogate decision-maker(s) (Zerwekh, 2006).

Use of Advance Directives

Studies show that although a majority of patients approve of ADs, the rate of completion of individual ADs is much lower (Johns, 1996). A study supported by the Agency for Healthcare Research and Quality (AHRQ) shows that ADs were in the medical records of less than 50% of severely or terminally ill patients in the sample. Another study reported that only 12% of patients with ADs had a conversation with their physicians about it (Kass-Bartelmes, Hughes, & Rutherford, 2003). A study by Valente (2004) indicated that clinicians in hospitals followed ADs for hospital treatment in 5% to 25% of end-of-life care situations.

Pediatric Patients

Although most state AD laws do not include children, the intent of ADs is applicable to children with decision-making capacity (Levetown, 2006). The Bioethics Committee of the American Academy of Pediatrics has developed guidelines for categories of medical orders. The "first order" means that no specified limits on therapy exist, and children will receive all medical interventions that are appropriate, including CPR. The "second order" means treatment such as CPR, intubation, or ventilation may be limited, when documented by physicians (Tan, Totapally, Torbati, & Wolfsdorf, 2006).

"Surrogates indicated that knowing patients' preferences for not being kept alive in certain conditions was the most important factor for help in decision-making."

End-of-life decision-making for pediatric patients has the added complexity of the parent-child relationship. In situations where a child is determined to have decision-making capacity, it may be difficult to honor those preferences and earlier decisions. Parents may experience guilt and a lack of readiness to follow through with decisions to limit treatment. They may believe they have failed as a parent if they let their child go, given their role of being the child's protector. In addition, they may misunderstand what life-sustaining treatment will do for their child. Hearing the words that their child is "stable" may be interpreted as the child will be okay (Levetown, 2006).

Surrogate Knowledge of Advance Directives

Many patients discuss end-of-life care in generalities with their family members. Hines et al. (2001) found that both patients and surrogates often overestimate the amount of knowledge the surrogate has about the patient's preferences. Surrogates indicated that knowing patients' preferences for not being kept alive in certain conditions was the most important factor for help in decision-making. The researchers concluded, however, that health professionals cannot determine that family members who have spoken with patients about treatment options will be knowledgeable surrogates in end-of-life decision-making.

Barriers to and Facilitators for Completing Advance Directives

Although health care organizations are required to talk to patients about whether an AD has been completed, many barriers interfere with actual completion of ADs. Patients may be reluctant to pursue AD completion for a variety of reasons. Patients may find it difficult to discuss end-of-life care with family members because of fear of disagreements among family members, concern about hurting those who were not selected as a health care proxy, and not wanting family members to suffer or be exposed to indignity at the end of life (Soskis, 1997). As discussed in Chapter 8, cultural beliefs can interfere with the desire to complete an AD. Patients may be influenced by overestimating their chance of recovery or having fear that they may regret completion of an AD.

Barriers to completion of ADs also result from the fears and concerns of health care professionals. These barriers include legal concerns, lack of knowledge about laws concerning ADs, and lack of education about how to discuss AD completion. Health professionals may fear discussing bad news and that AD completion will lead to suffering or conflict. Some health professionals see death as an enemy and believe that discussing AD completion implies giving in to death (Larson & Tobin, 2000).

What factors promote AD completion? Gauthier (2005) conducted in-depth interviews with 14 participants who were receiving hospice services to explore what influenced their end-of-life decision-making. Factors that increased their readiness for decision-making were worsening physical function, increasing physical pain, and increasing physical dependence. Strategies to enhance discussion of ADs included giving patients time to talk about what was important to them, initiating discussion early, and increasing health professional comfort with discussion through education and completion of a personal AD (Soskis, 1997). Some have suggested that one of the most caring and loving actions one can offer to the family is to have an honest discussion about decision-making for end-of-life health care (Ingalls, 2007; Perrin, 2006; Weaver, 2004).

The Nursing Role in Advance Care Planning Discussion

Although nurses have frequent opportunity for end-of-life discussions because of their proximity and frequent contact with patients, they may lack the knowledge and skills to be effective facilitators of discussion with patients and families. A survey of nursing personnel, mostly nurses, in two acute care facilities in Texas who had involvement with ADs indicated that participants lacked knowledge about the PSDA, ADs, and state law about ADs (Duke & Thompson, 2007). This knowledge gap can be addressed by developing strategies and tools for nurses to use to facilitate end-of-life discussion.

Nurses can be proactive in encouraging discussion on advance care planning in a way that invites patients into the decision-making process. See sidebar, "Nursing Interventions for Facilitating Advance Care Planning." In many of these interventions, listening and helping patients to reflect on what is important to them is foundational to the intervention.

Nursing Interventions for Facilitating Advance Care Planning

* Introduce ADs in primary care settings, such as during routine health exams and in ambulatory, noncrisis situations (Carney & Morrison, 1997; Maxfield, Pohl, & Colling, 2003).

* Approach end-of-life discussion in stages by moving from discussing who to include in decision-making to more difficult discussion about use of specific treatments at the end of life (Hines et al., 2001).

* Encourage choice through truth telling about positive and negative aspects, emphasizing the possibility of choice, translating medical information into human experience, asking questions to clarify options, and respecting the decision not to choose (Zerwekh, 2006, p. 187).

* Encourage patients and surrogates to determine how much freedom the surrogate should use in decision-making (Hines et al., 2001).

* Encourage patients and surrogates to discuss possible values conflicts about responding to situations of suffering and uncertainty (Hines et al., 2001).

* Encourage patients to customize their statements of preferences on advance directive documents (Ingalls, 2007).

* Recognize that you are working with a family unit (Ingalls, 2007).

* When discussing a DNR order, avoid asking, "Do you want everything done?" Many nonhealth professionals assume this includes provision of comfort, care, and support (Perrin, 2006).

* Suggest the following questions for family members to ask physicians to help them understand a patient's prognosis:

  * Based on your experience, how have you seen cases like this progress?

  * Is he or she going to recognize family members? Talk? Eat? Go to the bathroom on his or her own? (Ingalls, 2007)

- Avoid judging decisions and responses of patient and family (Ingalls, 2007).
- Refer to a social worker or chaplain when indicated for complex family dynamics and resource needs (Ingalls, 2007).

Advance Care Planning Programs and Models

Advance Care Planning programs and models indicate a structure for early decision-making with emphasis on decisional capacity for patients, explanations of how decision-making follows the illness trajectory, and strategies for patient- and health professional-initiated discussion about end-of-life choices.

Patient-Initiated Models of Advance Care Planning

Baines (2003) explains the use of ethical wills. "Ethical wills are a way to share your values, beliefs, life lessons, hopes for the future, love, and forgiveness with your family and community" (p. 141). Thoughts about end-of-life decisions may occur during life transitions such as marriage, birth of a child, birth of a grandchild, or retirement. Also, a significant life event such as serious illness, surgery, or loss of a family member or friend may lead to reflection about end-of-life choices (Baines, 2003). These reflections can provide an impetus for writing an ethical will. An outline for ethical wills has the following components:

- values and beliefs,
- knowledge and learning,
- giving and receiving,
- life lessons,
- hopes for the future, and
- concluding thoughts.

Guided writing exercises that begin with prompts such as "I am grateful for . . ." or "From my parents, I learned . . ." are also helpful for writing an ethical will. Examples of ethical wills are available at www.ethicalwill.com.

Five Wishes is a set of questions promoted by Aging with Dignity (2007), a national nonprofit organization (www.agingwithdignity.org/5wishes.html). These five questions guide people through expressing preferences for desired health care treatment at the end of life.

The Five Wishes

1. Which person do you want to make health care decisions for you when you can't make them?

2. What kind of medical treatment do you want or do you not want?

3. How comfortable do you want to be?

4. How do you want people to treat you?

5. What do you want your loved ones to know?

In 2007, Five Wishes was consistent with the legal requirements for advance directives in 40 U.S. states.

Clinical Models of Advance Care Planning

Larson and Tobin (2000) suggested a framework for initiating end-of-life discussions that considers illness progression and modification of health care goals. Although the model was created for a physician education program, the suggested actions and questions could be used by the interdisciplinary members of the health care team. See sidebar, "A Framework for Ongoing End-of-Life Discussions," for routine, structured, and ongoing end-of-life discussions.

Organizational and Community Models of Advance Care Planning

Gillick, Berkman, and Cullen (1999) described an advance care planning model for use in nursing homes. The patient and goal-centered approach was focused on prioritizing the goals of care as a guide to health care treatment choices at the end of

A Framework for Ongoing End-of-Life Discussions

1. Focus on a patient's experience of illness and how the patient makes decisions by making statements or asking questions such as the following:

   - Tell me about your illness.

   - What do you understand about your treatment options?

   - What are some of your concerns?

2. Help a patient to confront fears and take control by asking

   - What are your worried about or afraid of?

   - Have you lost family members or loved ones? How did they die, and what was it like for you?

3. Address practical issues such as advance care planning and family communication by asking

   - What problems is your illness creating for you?

   - Do any other loved ones or family members need to know what's going on?

4. Shift to a palliative care focus when indicated by the illness trajectory.

   - For example, say to patients, "There is a lot I can do for you at this time to control your pain, keep you comfortable, and help you live each day to the fullest extent you can."

5. Help patients achieve a peaceful and dignified death.

   - Say something like the following: "Sometimes people want to be sure to say goodbye to the people they love. If that is something you need to do, how might you do that?"

   - Ask the following: "Are there any unfinished parts of your life that you want to complete?"

Source: Larson & Tobin, 2000, pp. 1574-1575

life. The model is complex but comes closer to meeting the intent of advance directives to ensure that a patient's preferences are followed. Three possible goals—prolonging life, maintaining physical and cognitive function, and maximizing comfort—are ranked to determine a care pattern:

- Intensive pattern—prolonging life is the most important.

- Comprehensive care—maintaining physical and cognitive function is most important.

- Basic care—comfort is more important than prolonging life.

- Palliative care—comfort is most important, and maintaining physical and cognitive function is more important than prolonging life.

- Comfort only—the goal is to maximize comfort.

In an evaluation of the use of the goal-centered model with 38 nursing home residents and their surrogates, Gillick et al. (1999) found that the fewest choices were in the comfort-only category, and that rankings between patients and surrogates differed, with patients desiring more aggressive care.

Respecting Choices is an advance care planning program developed at Gunderson Lutheran Medical Center in La Crosse, Wisconsin (Briggs, 2003; Schwartz et al., 2002). In this comprehensive program, health care professionals and leaders at organizational and community levels intervene to change the culture around discussing death and dying. Strategies include facilitated discussions with patients and family about what patients want for end-of-life care and the benefits and burdens of treatment, as well as community-wide outreach to bring educational presentations to the relevant groups. LifeCare Conversations Collaborative (LCC) adapted the Respecting Choices model in Massachusetts to develop connections and linkages among community stakeholders for the purpose of creating a consensus and shared strategies for promoting end-of-life decision-making (Okun, 2003). LCC elements include "train the trainer" education; use of real-life scenarios to initiate ACP discussion; and use of "green sleeves," plastic sleeves to be placed on refrigerators for holding ADs. Both of these programs resulted in improvement in advance care planning processes in their communities.

Questions Nurses Can Ask to Promote Advance Care Planning

In addition to being good listeners, nurses need to develop the art of asking questions that help to assess the meaning of patients and families' experiences in end-of-life decision-making. The literature indicates many ideas for questions that help to explore beliefs, understanding, and meaning without being intrusive or offensive.

Questions to Ask in Advance Care Planning Discussion

For the Patient

- What activities or experiences are most important for your life at this time?

- What would make this time most meaningful for you?

- What are your thoughts about what health care you would like if you become sicker and closer to death?

- If you die unexpectedly, do you want heroic measures such as CPR to keep you alive?

Source: Dahlin & Giansiracusa, 2006

For the Family

- If the patient could wake up for 15 minutes and understand his or her condition fully, and then had to return to it, what would he or she tell you to do? (Quill, 2005, p. 1632)

For Parents

- Please tell me in your own words what you understand about your child's condition.

- How have you been involved in decision-making about your child's care up to this point? How have you felt about that involvement? How would you like to be involved?

- What are your wishes about the care being provided to your child?

- If you were looking at a time when your child may not be able to get through the illness, can you tell me what some of your wishes would be about that time? How would you like things to be?

- What are the most difficult things you are facing at this time? What do you think you might need to help you get through this time?

- Is there something you can think of that would help your child through this time?

Source: Levetown, 2006, p. 928

"If I could no longer make decisions for myself, what would I want to communicate to my family or to my health care providers?"

Reflective Practice

An advance care planning discussion is one of the most important communications that we can have with our patients and families as they approach end of life. This conversation should be dynamic and fluid. Wants and goals change as conditions change.

One of the best ways to prepare for this discussion is to complete your own advance directive. Ask yourself, "If I could no longer make decisions for myself, what would I want to communicate to my family or to my health care providers?"

Consider the directive on the next page completed by a nurse with many years of hospice experience

Keep in mind that although a written advance directive is a desired end product of these discussions, the discussion itself should be intentionally focused on exploring values, beliefs, and needs of patients and families about the kind of health care they would like to have at the end of life. We can emphasize the benefits of such discussion and making decisions—the patient is more likely to have the health care that is preferred, family members are more likely to know what the patient wants, patients will be less likely to suffer from aggressive care that does not help, and the burden of decision-making will be reduced for family members. End-of-life discussion can be framed as a gift.

These are my instructions to help guide my health care agent and my family in making care decisions, if I am unable to make them for myself.

❖ If I am unable to speak for myself and considered to be
   ___ In a terminal condition
   ___ In a coma with little hope of recovery
   ___ In a persistent vegetative state
   ___ Suffering from advanced dementia

❖ Then I want
   ___ Care that supports my comfort
   ___ Management of pain and other distressing physical symptoms
   ___ Hospice care at home if possible and acceptable to my family
   ___ Support for my family in honoring my wishes

❖ I do not want:
   ___ Feeding tubes, artificial nutrition, and hydration to prolong my life
   ___ Tests, procedures, or other treatments that will not add to my comfort or quality of my life
   ___ Resuscitation or intubation, except for the short-term purpose of organ donation
   ___ My care to place an extreme financial or caregiving burden on my family or my community

Furthermore, if I am unable to make and communicate my own decisions, and my health care agent decides it is in the best interests of my family and me to deviate from what is stated here, I give him full and final authority to do so.

_____   _____
Patient Signature   Date

Ethical Practice to Honor Advance Directives

ETHICAL PROBLEM: What should I do when advance directives are in the chart, but not being followed?

What Should I Value?

- Avoiding suffering for patient and family.
- Informed decision-making.
- Patient and family choice.
- Patient and family beliefs and values.
- Education about end-of-life choices.
- Quality end-of-life care.

Who Should I Be?

- A proactive advocate for the patient.
- A leader and change agent.
- Someone who seeks the evidence on effective care models and resources for advance care planning and advance directives.
- An effective interdisciplinary collaborator.

What Should I Do?

- Discuss the advance directive with the family.
- Engage physicians and the health care team in a discussion of the contents of the AD.
- Work with nurse managers, clinical educators, and colleagues to develop education and protocols for honoring advance directives.
- Request a consult from the ethics committee if conflicts exist.

Nurses' Stories

Advance Care Planning Versus Advance Directives

Because we work in health care, it is easy to become focused solely on treatment decisions. Advance directives help us address many of the treatment decisions, but are only part of an advance care planning discussion. A home care nurse tells about an experience she had in a class on advance directives:

I met another nurse in a continuing education class for nurses on advance directives. She told me she was writing hers and that it was already 25 pages long. She told me she worked in a nursing home and had seen a lot of her patients die. She didn't want the things that happened to them to happen to her, so she was trying to cover every possible scenario. The instructor asked her if she had discussed this with her family. She said, "No, because they wouldn't agree with me." The instructor then pointed out that in the event her directive was needed, her family would probably be asked to make the decisions. The instructor strongly encouraged the nursing home nurse to have a serious discussion with her family about what was important to her, rather than trying to write everything down.

Clarification and Understanding

Too often, especially in acute care settings, treatment decisions are made in the heat of the moment without finding out from patients or families what they understand about those decisions. A hospital palliative care nurse talks about the process of clarification with a little humor thrown in:

I had this woman with aspiration pneumonia. She had ataxia and aphasia. She was going to continue to aspirate. This was her fourth hospital admission in 3 months. She had the best sense of humor. After a discussion of code status and goals, she was still kind of confused. Her son said, "Mom it comes down to this, do you want to have a painful, horrible dying experience or do you want to be peaceful and comfortable? Do you want suffering or peace?" She looked at me and said, "I guess I want hospice."

Cultural Considerations

Patients and families from cultural backgrounds that base decision-making on values other than individual autonomy struggle with decisions they might be asked to make in end-of-life care. A nurse working with a sub-Saharan African family described the patient's confusion when asked about her treatment wishes:

We're asking people to make decisions on things they don't understand. We had a Somali woman who said, "Didn't that doctor go to medical school? Why is he asking me?"

Advance Care Planning and Directives With Children

Children represent a very special population concerning discussions about care wishes and goals at the end of life. With children, advance directives are not legal, because a child cannot be the legal decision-maker. All decisions fall on the parents. A children's palliative care nurse talks about her approach—especially with babies:

> With kids, advance directives aren't legal. We approach it by asking parents to look at themselves, because these are the values they raise their children with. We ask, "What are your family values?" and [we] help them see it from their point of view. Because with babies, that's what you do.

Key Points

- Advance care planning is a thoughtful discussion about care wishes and goals at the end of life.

- Advance directives are legal documents expressing treatment preferences when people can no longer speak for themselves.

- Nurses play a significant role in facilitating discussions about end-of-life goals.

- Many care models exist that nurses can use to facilitate these discussions.

REFLECTION QUESTIONS

1. What kinds of discussions have you had with family members or patients and their family members about planning for end-of-life care?

2. What are some conversation-openers that you would feel comfortable using in introducing end-of-life care planning to patients and families?

3. In your health care organization, what are the practices for advance care planning? When are advance directives discussed? How do you think the practice of promoting advance care planning could be improved in your organization?

Tools and Resources for Facilitating Advance Care Planning

Advance Care Planning Admission Assessment

Briggs, L., & Colvin, E. (2002). The nurse's role in end-of life decision-making for patients and families. *Geriatric Nursing, 23*(6), 302-310.

Advance Directives (AARP)

http://www.aarp.org/research/legal/advancedirect/

American Bar Association: Health Care Advance Directives

http://www.abanet.org/publiced/practical/healthcare_directives.html

Booklet for Patients and Families on CPR, Artificial Feeding, and Comfort Care

Dunn, H. (2001). *Hard choices for loving people.* Herndon, VA: A & A Publishers. Retrieved April 20, 2009, at www.hardchoices.com

Decision Tree for Nurses

http://www2.edc.org/lastacts/archives/archivesJan99/decisiontree.asp

Download Your State's Advance Directives

http://www.caringinfo.org/stateaddownload

Innovations in End-of-Life Care Resources and Tools

http://www2.edc.org/lastacts/archives/archivesMay03/resources.asp

Questionnaire on Information and Decision-Making Preferences

Gauthier, D. M., & Froman, R. D. (2001). Preferences for care near the end of life: Scale development and validation. *Research in Nursing & Health, 24,* 298-306.

Murtagh, F. E. M., & Thorns, A. (2006). Evaluation and ethical review of a tool to explore patient preferences for information and involvement in decision-making. *Journal of Medical Ethics, 32,* 311-315.

Respecting Choices Tools and Website Links

http://www2.edc.org/lastacts/archives/archivesJan99/resources.asp

References

Aging with Dignity. (2007*). Five wishes.* Retrieved September 30, 2008, from www.agingwithdignity.org/5wishes.html

Baines, B. K. (2003). Ethical wills: Creating meaning at the end of life. *Home Health Care Management & Practice, 15*(2), 140-146.

Briggs, L. (2003). Shifting the focus of advance care planning: Using an in-depth interview to build and strengthen relationships. *Innovations in End-of-Life Care, 5*(2). Retrieved April 20, 2009, from http://www2.edc.org/lastacts/archives/archivesMarch03/default.asp

Carney, M., & Morrison, R. (1997). Advance directives: When, why, and how to start talking. *Geriatrics, 52,* 65-72.

Dahlin, C. M., & Giansiracusa, D. F. (2006). Communication in palliative care. In B. R. Ferrell & N. Coyle, (Eds.), *Textbook of palliative care nursing* (pp. 67-93). New York: Oxford University Press.

Duke, G., Thompson, S., & Hastie, M. (2007). Factors influencing completion of advanced directives in hospitalized patients. *International Journal of Palliative Nursing, 13*(1), 39-43.

Dunn, H. (2001). *Hard choices for loving people.* Herndon, VA: A & A Publishers. Retrieved April 20, 2009, at http://www.hardchoices.com

Gauthier, D. M. (2005). Decision making near the end of life. *Journal of Hospice and Palliative Nursing, 7*(2), 82-90.

Gauthier, D. M., & Froman, R. D. (2001). Preferences for care near the end of life: Scale development and validation. *Research in Nursing & Health, 24,* 298-306.

Gillick, M., Berkman, S., & Cullen, L. (1999). A patient-centered approach to advance planning in the nursing home. *Journal of the American Geriatrics Society, 47*(2), 227-230.

Hines, S. C., Glover, J. J., Babrow, A. S., Holley, J. L., Badzek, L. A., & Moss, A. H. (2001). Improving advance care planning by accommodating family preferences. *Journal of Palliative Medicine, 4*(4), 481-489.

Ingalls, L. (2007). Bring your love: Therapeutic and effective end-of-life discussions. *Home Health Care Management & Practice, 19*(5), 369-381.

Johns, J. L. (1996). Advance directives and opportunities for nurses. *Image: Journal of Nursing Scholarship, 28*(2), 149-153.

Kass-Bartelmes, B. L., Hughes, R., & Rutherford, M. K. (2003). *Advance care planning: Preferences for care at the end of life.* Rockville, MD: Agency for Healthcare Research and Quality. Research in Action Issue #12. AHRQ Pub No. 03-0018.

Larson, D. G., & Tobin, D. R. (2000). End-of-life conversations: Evolving practice and theory. *JAMA, 284*(12), 1573-1578.

Levetown, M. (2006). Pediatric care: Transitioning goals of care in the emergency department, intensive care unit, and in between. In B. R. Ferrell & N. Coyle, (Eds.), *Textbook of palliative care nursing* (pp. 925-943). New York: Oxford University Press.

Matzo, M. L., & Ramsey, G. C. (2006). Legal aspects of end-of-life care. In M. L. Matzo & D. W. Sherman (Eds.), *Palliative care nursing* (pp. 187-217.). New York: Springer.

Maxfield, C. L., Pohl, J. M., & Colling, K. (2003). Advance directives: A guide for patient discussions. The *Nurse Practitioner, 28*(5), 38-47.

Moore, C. D. (2005). Communication issues and advance care planning. *Seminars in Oncology Nursing, 21*(1), 11-19.

Norlander, L., & McSteen, K. (2000). The kitchen table discussion: A creative way to discuss end-of-life issues. *Home Healthcare Nurse, 18*(8), 532-539.

Okun, S. (2003). A framework for collaborative consumer-oriented care. *Innovations in End-of-Life Care, 5*(3). Retrieved April 20, 2009, from http://www2.edc.org/lastacts/archives/archivesMay03/default.asp

Pearlman, R. A., Cole, W. G., Patrick, D. L., Starks, H. E., & Cain, K. C. (1995). Advance care planning: Eliciting patient preferences for life-sustaining treatment. *Patient Education and Counseling, 26*, 532-539.

Perrin, K. O. (2006). Communicating with seriously ill and dying patients, their families, and their health care providers. In M. L. Matzo & D. W. Sherman (Eds.), *Palliative care nursing* (pp. 221-245). New York: Springer.

Quill, T. (2005). Terri Schiavo—A tragedy compounded. *New England Journal of Medicine, 352*(16), 1630-1632.

Schwartz, C. E., Wheeler, H. B., Hammes, B., Basque, N., Edmunds, J., Reed, G., et al. (2002). Early intervention in planning end-of-life care with ambulatory geriatric patients. *Archives of Internal Medicine, 162*, 1611-1618.

Soskis, C. W. (1997). End-of-life decisions in the home care setting. *Social Work in Health Care, 25*(1/2), 107-116.

Tan, G. H., Totapally, B. R., Torbati, D., & Wolfsdorf, J. (2006). End-of-life decisions and palliative care in a children's hospital. *Journal of Palliative Medicine, 9*(2), 332-342.

Valente, S. M. (2004). End-of-life challenges: Honoring autonomy. *Cancer Nursing, 27*(4), 314-319.

Weaver, A. W. (2004). Family health promotion during life-threatening illness at the end of life. In P. T. Bomar (Ed.), *Promoting health in families: Applying family research and theory to nursing practice* (pp. 507-533). Philadelphia: Saunders.

Zerwehk, J. V. (2006). *Nursing care at the end of life.* Philadelphia: F. A. Davis.

I received a call from the very distraught son of a woman with advanced dementia. She'd been in a nursing home for more than 10 years and was now pushing away food. The nursing home [staff] was tying her hands down and trying to spoon feed her. He wanted them to stop, but they said they couldn't because she would starve to death. He was frantic because he said that before his mother got so sick, she had told him she didn't want to be kept alive if she couldn't eat. He thought his mother was communicating her wishes by pushing the food away. We helped the son transfer the patient to another facility where they would honor his wish that they offer her food and if she chose to eat it, fine, but if not, they wouldn't force it on her. She slowly declined to eat and died peacefully on our hospice program 2 months later. I think about that patient when people tell me, "The patients can't tell us what they want." I believe that she did communicate with us.

–Hospice Nurse

10

•

Challenges in End-of-Life Communication

Communication with patients, families, and health care providers is the key to ensuring good end-of-life care. Often, however, we are working with challenging populations and complex health care environments. How do you determine the wishes and goals of patients with advanced dementia or cognitive disability? How do you approach those who are homeless or disenfranchised from the mainstream? What about children and their rights and ability to decide their own care?

Determination of Ability to Make Decisions

Two terms are used to address the ability to make decisions—*capacity* and *competency*. Although both terms have to do with making a rational decision, competency is the legal term and is determined by the court. Decisional capacity, on the other hand, is determined through clinical assessment (Matzo & Ramsey, 2006; Zerwekh, 2006). The American Medical Directors Association (2006) provides a framework for assessing capacity to make health care decisions and offers several guidelines for working through the determination of capacity for health care decision-making:

- Look for consistent responses to questions that are phrased differently.

- Consider that information may be better understood with the use of visual aids.

- Address psychological issues and promote family support to improve capacity to make decisions.

- Ensure that choices offered to patients who are mentally incapacitated do not involve risks to their health through unwise choices.

- Balance the risks of poor decisions with the loss of autonomy.

- Can the person express personal preferences?

Assessing Decisional Capacity

- Can the person give reasons for any choices expressed?
- Do the reasons flow logically from the discussion and information provided?
- Can the person give the possible risks and benefits of choices that are consistent with the discussion?
- Can the person identify what is important to him or her, and does the choice reflect his or her values?

Sources: American Medical Directors Association, 2006; Zerwekh, 2006

Consensus Approach to Health Care Decisions

The major rationale for assessing decision-making capacity is to protect patients from unsafe decisions (Zerwekh, 2006). Berrie and Griffie (2006) suggest that a consensus approach is best for patients who are unable to make safe decisions. As an alternative to following a decision-making hierarchy, a consensus approach ensures the consideration of a greater amount of information provided by the variety of stakeholders involved in the end-of-life care situation, and increases the likelihood that a decision will be based on both knowledge of patients' conditions and their desires and values. A consensus approach to decision-making may also take more time and generate some tension as different views are expressed.

Conflicts of Interest

Swedish researchers Bolmsjo and Hermeren (2003) conducted a study on conflicts of interest encountered in the experiences of family members of relatives with amyotrophic lateral sclerosis (ALS). In their discussion, the researchers suggest situations in which it is ethically justifiable to override the wishes of patients or family members:

- The patient is temporarily confused or permanently incompetent.

- Patients or family members do not understand the best interests of one another.

- Patients or family members have misunderstood the information given by the physician.

- Patients or family members have incorrectly balanced the interests of the different stakeholders involved.

An open and *transparent* dialogue will help to identify the facts, conflict of values or interests and preferences, and the consequences and benefits of possible decisions. Bolsmsjo and Hermeren (2003) suggested that dialogue may result in changing unfounded beliefs and can also give insight to determine whether a situation justifies overriding the wishes of the patient or family. The legal mandates of the state or country in which the situation occurs are important to consider when analyzing the benefits and consequences of overriding patient or family decisions. The overall goal is to reduce potential harm to patients.

Dementia and End-of-Life Communication

It is estimated that 50% to 75% of nursing home residents have dementia (Magaziner, Zimmerman, Fox, & Burns, 1998). Dementia is considered to be a progressive, terminal illness without cure, but it has an uncertain illness trajectory; some people may live 20 years after the diagnosis (Lloyd-Williams & Payne, 2002; Powers & Watson, 2008).

"End-of-life decision-making about health care choices for patients with dementia can be an arduous journey for families."

End-of-life decision-making about health care choices for patients with dementia can be an arduous journey for families. Forbes, Bern-Klug, and Gessert (2000) conducted focus groups in four racially and economically diverse nursing homes to explore decision-making processes of family members about end-of-life treatments. They identified five themes that describe the decision-making experiences of family members of patients with severe dementia:

* Decision-making is emotionally difficult and involves burden, guilt, and sense of responsibility.

* Dementia is an "insult to life," because dementia changes the personhood of residents and results in a loss of relationships.

* There are two views of death with dementia—tragedy or blessing. Family members struggle with framing the death of a loved one with dementia as either a tragedy or a blessing.

* Values and goals surrounding end-of-life treatments are part of the context of decision-making. Comfort for the patient and peace of mind for the family member were goals identified by focus group participants. However, few participants were able to translate the goal of comfort to care choices that led to a natural death for residents. Decision-making is complex because "peace of mind" may be understood as "doing everything that could be done," which is inconsistent with a natural death.

- The dying trajectory for patients with dementia is unrecognized. Although participants said they did not want to prolong suffering of their relatives, they felt compelled to treat what could be treated. They made decisions on a day-to-day or "in the moment" basis, rather than making decisions from a "big picture" perspective. Examples of decisions included whether hospitalization or aggressive treatment was indicated for pneumonia and whether a feeding tube should be used when a patient lost the ability to swallow.

The findings of the Forbes et al. study indicate that nurses and other health care professionals can help family members through their difficult journey by discussing the trajectory of disease; exploring values and goals surrounding death and end-of-life treatment; and addressing confusion, burden, and guilt (Forbes et al., 2000). These communication interventions can help family members recognize "when the time has come" to move toward a natural and peaceful death as beneficial for both patients and families, and to realize what decisions were needed to accomplish that goal.

Communication Interventions for Patients With Dementia

- Look for nonverbal indicators of hunger, pain, or illness, such as facial expression, tense body language, or agitation (Ouldred & Bryant, 2008).

- Provide clear information to family members about the disease trajectory, complications of dementia, and treatment options (Ouldred & Bryant).

- Acknowledge emotions of family members and express caring and support for their experience (Caron, Griffith, & Arcand, 2005).

- Help family members discuss any guilt they experienced in making decisions (Caron et al.).

- Discuss family members' values about quality of life for their dying relative (Caron et al.).

- Collaborate with social workers on discussion of advance directives, and provide information about patients' status, dying trajectories, and treatment options and responses (Lacey, 2006).

Disenfranchised Patients at the End of Life

Disability

For dying patients who are intellectually disabled, the expected death may not be openly discussed or acknowledged, and they are often not included in decisions related to death, such as funeral planning (Read & Thompson, 2008). End-of-life decision-making for people with an intellectual disability is complicated by health professionals' lack of knowledge about intellectual disabilities, lack of understanding about laws regarding consent for treatment, and using personal standards and perspectives to judge someone else's quality of life. Accurate communication is hampered when individuals cannot explain their discomfort, express feelings in a sociable manner, or read health information. Communication is further hampered when staff cannot understand or interpret the discomfort of patients with intellectual disabilities (Read & Thompson).

End-of-Life Communication for Patients With a Cognitive Disability

- Look for assessment tools that measure distress for people with limited verbal and cognitive abilities.
    - Disability Distress Assessment Tool (DisDAT) http://www.crfr.ac.uk/disdat/Disdattool.pdf
    - Abbey Scale (Abbey et al., 2004)
- Allow adequate time for patients to understand what you are telling them about the illness.
- Use pictures along with words to promote understanding.
- Use simple sentences, and break them down into understandable pieces of information.
- Record discussions on audiotape, so patients can listen again.
- Respect patients' rights to make decisions and choices within the limitation of safe options that will not result in additional harm.
- Recognize your own skill deficits in working with patients with intellectual disabilities, and identify strategies to improve skills.

Source: Read & Thompson, 2008

Homelessness

Homeless people have a greater risk for a "bad death" because they often do not have an advance directive (AD) or an identified decision maker. Their episodic pattern of health care may lead to futile life-saving treatment that contributes to greater suffering and prevents a peaceful death (Hughes, 2006). Kushel and Miaskowski (2006) suggest that homeless people are less likely to use hospice because of a lack of financial resources, social support, and a home base for needed hospice services. Negative experiences with the health care system may lead homeless people to believe that needed care will not be given. As survivors in a difficult life, they may request cardiopulmonary resuscitation (CPR) and aggressive treatment (Kushel & Miaskowski).

Ethical Practice in Providing End-of-Life Care to Homeless People

ETHICAL PROBLEM: What should I do when a homeless patient who is dying insists on receiving treatments that will not improve the status and will likely contribute to greater suffering?

What Should I Value?

* Patient preferences.
* A peaceful death experience.
* Relationship-centered care.
* Meeting the needs of all people who are dying.

Who Should I Be?

* A compassionate nurse who works to understand the perspectives and experiences of homeless people.
* A humble nurse who recognizes his or her own limitations and works to understand the reality of the situation of homeless people, including the struggle to survive.
* Knowledgeable about hospice and health care services for homeless populations.

What Should I Do?

* Seek education about effective communication strategies for working with homeless people.

- Listen to the stories of patients.
- Provide an explanation of likely outcomes of hospitalization for life-prolonging treatment.
- Offer other options for care that can support a peaceful death for patients.
- Advocate for a shelter-based care option through involvement in palliative program development for homeless people.

Results from focus group sessions with 20 homeless people at an urban health care clinic show insight about the participants' end-of-life experiences, their decision-making practices, and treatment preferences (Tarzian, Neal, & O'Neil, 2005). Five major themes from the analysis indicate participants' concerns about receiving less than optimal care:

1. Participants believed that end-of-life "wants" should be honored. Preferences ranged from wanting life prolonged to emphasis on high quality of life. Some participants were concerned about being undertreated related to discriminatory practices and viewed themselves as survivors who could "beat the odds."

2. Participants acknowledged the intensity of emotion in end-of-life experiences—the hurt involved in dealing with loss.

3. Religious beliefs and spiritual experiences were a core component of end-of-life experiences. Participants talked about an afterlife that would be free of the pain of the world. It was important to respect God's will and timing.

4. Participants wanted relationship-centered care—they wanted someone who was compassionate and who would listen to them, comfort them, and "keep hope alive."

5. Participants were ambivalent about advance care planning. They thought it was a good idea but were concerned about putting anything into writing—based on fears that they would receive less than optimal treat-

ment because of discrimination by health care providers and insurance companies. However, they also thought having something written could help the health care proxy make a decision without being burdened by feeling guilty that they had contributed to someone's death.

Based on these themes, the authors recommended that end-of-life care for homeless people should include advance care planning as a process rather than an end product, such as an AD. Shelter-based programs have the potential to provide the support homeless people need to make decisions that are more likely to result in a peaceful death. The Ottawa Inner City Health Project provides comprehensive health services to homeless adults (Podymow, Turnbull, & Coyle, 2006). An analysis of 28 homeless people who died at the shelter-based hospice revealed that most patients requested or agreed to a do-not-resuscitate order. Most agreed they would not want to be hospitalized, but rather wanted to die in a familiar place. Costs of care were less for the shelter-based palliative care program.

End-of-Life Care Communication for Homeless People

- Focus discussion on relationships and how family members and health care providers can help them with decision-making, rather than emphasizing individual autonomy.

- Work to understand the lived experiences of homeless people—listen to their stories.

- Facilitate expression of emotional and spiritual needs.

- Start conversations early before illness becomes terminal, and plan for multiple conversations to ensure understanding and build trust.

- Present a scenario of a hypothetical medical crisis to promote understanding.

- Ask what concerns they have about dying—experiences of family members and friends, and fears of dying alone or on the street.

- Plan for safekeeping of a completed AD—recommend that they carry their AD with them.

- Document patients' requests, along with emergency contact information.

Sources: Kushel & Miaskowski, 2006; Tarzian et al., 2005

Challenges With Parents and Children

End-of-life decision-making for children must also meet legal requirements for informed consent. Informed consent is consistent with supporting a patient's autonomy and requires disclosure, comprehension, voluntariness, competence, and consent (Veach, 2001). For parents and children, decision-making involves the autonomy of several individuals. One way to support a child's autonomy in the decision-making process is to obtain assent, when developmentally feasible. Assent is a legal concept that gives consideration to a child's understanding and opinions about health care choices. "By obtaining assent, a health care provider is ensuring that a child's decision is in agreement with the decision of the designated parent or legal guardian who will give informed consent" (Jacobs, 2005, p. 362). In some cases a child will need to receive treatments that they do not want because of parental and provider decision making. Nursing interventions in working with children and parents involve consideration of multiple perspectives—those of the parents, child, and interdisciplinary health care team members.

End-of-Life Care Communication for Children

- Ask children about what they want for health care to help determine goals and perceptions about burdens of care treatment.

- Involve siblings in the dying process, and refer them to a child development specialist if possible.

- Collaborate with family to incorporate cultural rituals and practices into care.

- Avoid use of the word "withdrawal," and emphasize what care *will* be given.

- Avoid being judgmental about a parent's refusal to withhold or withdraw medical interventions; refer complex, difficult situations to an ethics committee.

- Be proactive in planning. Work with the interdisciplinary health care team to determine goals of care pre-crisis, so that there is a common understanding between family and health care professionals about possible scenarios for withholding or withdrawing treatments.

- Encourage the parents to talk with their child about death; explain that parents are usually glad that they talked about death with their child (Kreicbergs, Valdimarsdottir, Oneslov, Henter, & Steineck, 2004).

Source: Jacobs, 2005

Scripts for End-of-Life Care

Providing effective end-of-life care is often challenged by set expectations or "scripts" in a health care setting. In critical care settings, cure is often the goal; life-saving technical skills and medical frameworks are usually emphasized (Pattison, 2004). For long-term care settings, the emphasis is on living; rehabilitation, maintenance, and prevention are the words of choice, not death and dying (Oliver, Porock, & Oliver, 2006). In addition, the scripts for hospice and palliative care are different and sometimes misunderstood. Powers and Watson (2008) provide clear definitions of hospice and palliative care:

- Hospice is "a care delivery system oriented toward comfort care of dying" (p. 324).

- Palliative care is "a holistic approach that is focused on relieving suffering and enhancing quality of life by coordinating provider efforts and tailoring care plans to patient-family goals and values" (p. 324).

Long-Term Care

A secondary analysis of interviews with 16 nursing home staff (RNs, LPNs, and social service workers) indicated the tension and conflict between the two scripts of the public message of rehabilitation and the private reality of death in a nursing home (Oliver et al., 2006). Staff members found they had no formal script or policy to help families with the death of a resident. Oliver and colleagues suggest that the palliative care script should be integrated into long-term care settings, and the public needs education to be aware of and accept the palliative care script.

Care of the dying should not be hidden; death is an expected outcome. Death does not mean that care is poor; instead, death is inevitable and a natural outcome of a physiological process. The *Guidelines of End-of-Life Care in Long-Term Care Facilities* is a good example of policy to make dying a front-stage script in long-term care settings (Missouri Department of Health and Senior Services, 2003).

"Changing the script to champion palliative care approaches in our current health care environment requires courage."

Lusk (2007) discusses the importance of meaningful relationships in the long-term care setting in which many staff members have "family-like" relationships or are surrogate family members for residents. However, it is also the direct care staff with the least education that has the greatest burden of care of dying patients. Communication difficulties, often stemming from a lack of education and understanding, can lead to additional suffering for patients and families, which also creates distress for staff.

Critical Care

When life can no longer be prolonged, a critical care script becomes ineffective and futile. Uncertainty about prognosis and outcomes makes decisions about when to stop treatment difficult. Pattison (2004) suggests that end-of-life care in critical care settings can be enhanced by integrating both the palliative and critical care paradigms (scripts), rather than seeing them as a dichotomy for patients who are at risk for dying. The focus needs to be on the patient's condition and the best response to his or her condition. In that way, interventions become holistic and serve the best interests of patients. Comfort is viewed as an important goal and is not compromised by having cure as the only goal.

Reflective Practice

Changing the script to champion palliative care approaches in our current health care environment requires courage. This is especially the case when working with patients who have impairments that make determining their wishes difficult. Our own discomfort and possible bias toward challenging patients, added to a lack of knowledge about how to effectively communicate with them, increase the complexity.

Imagine…

Step back and imagine yourself suffering from dementia, and every person who comes into your room is new to you. People are doing things to you that you don't understand, and you are frightened. How would you communicate with them? How would you like them to communicate with you?

In self-reflection, we become aware of our own strengths and weaknesses and acknowledge our biases and mistakes. By recognizing our own limitations, we also become more accepting of the limitations of others (Crigger, 2004). As humble people, we develop a realistic understanding of our own place in the world and our relationships and interconnectedness with others (de Vries, 2004). Humility makes possible an understanding of what we can and cannot do in challenging communication situations, yet it allows us to develop the connections necessary to do what we can do to improve quality of end-of-life care for patients who are dying.

Nurses' Stories

Cognitively Impaired Patients

Connecting with a patient who has advanced dementia or some other type of cognitive impairment requires the ability to look beyond verbal communication. A hospice nurse relates the case of a patient who became combative whenever anyone tried to touch her. Reviewing the case with her hospice team of a social worker, pharmacist, and team physician helped her to address the behavior and make the patient more comfortable.

> The patient couldn't say more than a few words. When she was by herself in her room, she seemed fine. But, when anyone tried to touch her or do [something] for her, she became agitated and batted people away. We couldn't figure out what it was until I presented the case in [a team meeting] and another nurse asked me, "Is she this way all the time?" And I said, "Only when someone tries to touch her." The other nurse said, "Maybe she's trying to tell you that she's in pain when she's reacting that way." We looked at

her medical history, and she had a neurological condition that could cause her pain upon [being touched]. The hospice doctor and pharmacist recommended a medication that could help that kind of pain. I wouldn't have figured it out without the help of the team.

Children at the End of Life

Dying children are especially vulnerable. Parents and families want to protect them. Health care professionals want to save them from dying. Sometimes in the midst of trying to do the best for a child, the child's voice gets lost. A pediatric palliative care nurse talks about her experience with a dying child:

She was a school-aged kid and everybody loved her. The physician and nurse practitioner who were treating her were kind of enmeshed. Our home care nurses went out and found that her pain and breathlessness were not under control. I called the nurse practitioner and she said, "Oh, the mom isn't a good historian, and I don't think there's a problem." She wouldn't give me a prescription. The little girl said she had pain, but when the nurse practitioner talked with the mom, the mom said everything is fine. The little girl wanted pain IVs so she wouldn't have to take pills. The last straw was when the little girl wrote a note to our home care nurse that said, "Help me, help me." We called the physician, and the doctor talked with her. They finally gave the order.

Mentally Ill Patients

Working with an interdisciplinary team when you have difficult patients can be crucial to seeing that patients receive the services they need. In this case, a nurse and social worker needed the help of outside resources.

We were seeing this elderly patient at home with severe cardiac disease. She lived alone, had no family, and had a long history of mental illness. She was distrustful and often would not let us come into the home. It was obvious, when we did see her, that she was getting worse, but she wouldn't take her medicines and she insisted, "I want to die at home, and I want everyone to leave me alone." We finally had to call Adult Protective Services, because she was so sick and she wouldn't let us help. They ended up taking

her to the hospital against her wishes, and that's where she died. This was
difficult for the care team, but sometimes we can't honor patient's wishes
when they aren't able to make good decisions.

Key Points

- Communication at the end of life is especially challenging when working with certain populations:

    - Those with dementia or with cognitive or intellectual impairment.

    - Those who are disenfranchised from the mainstream health care system, such as the homeless or mentally ill.

    - Children.

- Appropriate communication with these populations involves determining the capacity to make rational decisions. The concept of decisional capacity differs from decisional competency. *Competency* is a legal term determined by the court. *Capacity* is determined through clinical assessment.

- Recognize our own limitations and biases in accepting the limitations of others.

REFLECTION QUESTIONS

1. What communication strategies can you use to enhance communication with patients whose level of understanding and ability to communicate are challenged by dementia or disability?

2. What can nurses and the health care system do to improve communication in end-of-life care for homeless patients who are dying?

3. Explain the "script" for end-of-life care that is predominant in your work or learning setting. How do you think the "script" needs to be changed?

References

Abbey, J., Piller, N., DeBellis, A., Esterman, A., Parker, D., Giles, L. et al. (2004). The Abbey pain scale: A 1-minute numerical indicator for people with end-stage dementia. *International Journal of Palliative Nursing, 10*(1), 6-13.

American Medical Directors Association. (2003). White paper on surrogate decision-making and advance care planning in long-term care. Retrieved October 11, 2008, from http://www.amda.com/governance/whitepapers/surrogate/surrogate.pdf

Berrie, P., & Griffe, J. (2006). Planning for the actual death In B. R. Ferrell & N. Coyle (Eds.), *Textbook of palliative care nursing* (pp. 561-577). New York: Oxford University Press.

Bolmsjo, I., & Hermeren, G. (2003). Conflicts of interest: Experiences of close relatives of patients suffering from amyotrophic lateral sclerosis. *Nursing Ethics, 10*(2), 187-198.

Caron, C. D., Griffith, J., & Arcand, M. (2005). End-of-life decision making in dementia: A perspective of family caregivers. *Dementia, 4*(1), 113-136.

Crigger, N. J. (2004). Always having to say you're sorry: An ethical response to making mistakes in professional practice. *Nursing Ethics, 11*, 568-576.

de Vries, K. (2004). Humility and its practice in nursing. *Nursing Ethics, 11*, 77-586.

Forbes, S., Bern-Klug, M., & Gessert, C. (2000). End-of-life decision making for nursing home residents with dementia. *Journal of Nursing Scholarship, 32*(3), 251-258.

Hughes, A. (2006). Poor, homeless, and underserved populations. In B. R. Ferrell & N. Coyle (Eds.), *Textbook of palliative nursing* (pp. 661-670). New York: Oxford University Press.

Jacobs, H. H. (2005). Ethics in pediatric end-of-life care. *Journal of Pediatric Nursing, 20*(5), 360-369.

Kreicbergs, U., Valdimarsdottir, U., Oneslov, E., Henter, J. I., & Steineck, G. (2004). Talking with children who have severe malignant disease. *New England Journal of Medicine, 35*(12), pp. 1175-1186.

Kushel, M. B., & Miaskowski, C. (2006). End-of-life care for homeless patients. *JAMA, 296*(24), 2959-2966.

Lacey, D. (2006). End-of-life decision making for nursing home residents with dementia: A survey of nursing home social services staff. *Health & Social Work, 31*(3), 189-199.

Lloyd-Williams, M., & Payne, S. (2002). Can multidisciplinary guidelines improve the palliation of symptoms in the terminal phase of dementia? *International Journal of Palliative Nursing, 8*(8), 370-375.

Lusk, C. (2007). The need for palliative/end-of-life programs in LTC. *Canadian Nursing Home, 18*(4), 9-15.

Magaziner, J., Zimmerman, S. I., Fox, K. M., & Burns, B. J. (1998). Dementia in United States nursing homes: Descriptive epidemiology and implications for long-term residential care. *Aging and Mental Health, 2,* 28-35.

Matzo, M. L., & Ramsey, G. C. (2006). Legal aspects of end-of-life care. In M. L. Matzo & D. W. Sherman (Eds.), *Palliative care nursing* (pp. 187-217). New York: Springer.

Missouri Department of Health and Senior Services. (2003). *Guidelines of end-of-life care in long-term care facilities: With emphasis on developing palliative care goals.* Jefferson City, MO: Author.

Oliver, D. P., Porock, D., & Oliver, D. B. (2006). Managing the secrets of dying backstage: The voices of nursing home staff. *OMEGA, 53*(3), 193-207.

Ouldred, E., & Bryant, C. (2008). Dementia care. Part 3: End-of-life care for people with advanced dementia. *British Journal of Nursing, 17*(5), 308-314.

Pattison, N. (2004). Integration of critical care and palliative care at the end of life. *British Journal of Nursing, 13*(3), 132-139.

Podymow, T., Turnbull, J., & Coyle, D. (2006). Shelter-based palliative care for the homeless terminally ill. *Palliative Medicine, 20,* 81-86.

Powers, B. A., & Watson, N. M. (2008). Meaning and practice of palliative care for nursing home residents with dementia at end of life. *American Journal of Alzheimer's Disease and Other Dementias, 23*(4), 319-325.

Read, S., & Thompson-Hill, J. (2008). Palliative care nursing in relation to people with intellectual disabilities. *British Journal of Nursing, 17*(8), 506-510.

Tarzian, A. J., Neal, M. T., & O'Neil, J. A. (2005). Attitudes, experiences, and beliefs affecting end-of-life decision-making among homeless individuals. *Journal of Palliative Medicine, 8*(1), 36-48.

Veach, R. M. (Ed.). (2001). *Medical ethics.* Sudbury, MA: Jones and Bartlett.

Zerwekh, J. V. (2006). *Nursing care at the end of life.* Philadelphia: F. A. Davis.

We have a ceremony at the beginning of each team meeting where we can put a stone in the water for patients we've lost and say something about them. This is the time when we talk about the real people behind the symptoms and all the messy medical stuff. This is the time when we talk about how they touched our lives, and this is why I work in hospice.

—Hospice nurse

11

•

Taking Care of
Yourself

Being present for our patients and families during life's final journey can be stressful and draining. It can also be one of the richest experiences a nurse can have. How we balance the difficult work with its many rewards affects how we care for our patients. Understanding the stressors and practicing self-care are key to the balance.

Sources of Stress in End-of-Life Care

Stress is about perception. Individuals perceive stress when they have conflict between what they would like to have happen or think should happen and what is actually happening. In palliative care, nurses may experience stress from role strain when they cannot adequately perform their nursing role as expected because of lack of education, experience, or ability (Babant, 2001). Some sources of stress for palliative care nurses, such as workload pressures and relationships with other health professionals, are similar to stressors experienced by nurses in all care specialties. The effect of the sadness of patients and families is an additional stressor identified in interviews with community palliative care nurses in the United Kingdom (Newton & Waters, 2001). End-of-life care challenges that contributed to stress for the nurses in the study were over-identification with the patient and family, having their skills tested by symptoms or difficult situations they could not control, being prevented from providing optimum care, and an accumulation of sadness that contributed to feelings of vulnerability.

"Feelings of inadequacy and the belief that the situation will not change contribute to decreased enthusiasm for work, job dissatisfaction, lack of confidence, and distrust in the organization."

Newton and Walters (2001) described the possibility of an overwork stress spiral resulting from workload pressures, such as a constant stream of referrals with inadequate time for accomplishing the workload. Feelings of inadequacy and the belief that the situation will not change contribute to decreased enthusiasm for work, job dissatisfaction, lack of confidence, and distrust in the organization. If the stress spiral continues, a nurse may become ill or experience problems at home, and may choose to leave the job.

Bruce (2008) explored the emotional work of palliative care nurses and physicians in the interprofessional environment of palliative care. Although study participants described their work as meaningful and found the palliative care philosophy consistent with their values and beliefs, they also experienced stressors from emotional challenges in their work. The analysis indicated the following themes concerning emotional challenges:

- Working on interdisciplinary teams could be both rewarding and distressing. Disagreements and physician-controlled work led to frustrations.

- Participants viewed end-of-life care as emotional and personal work. They viewed self-awareness and reflection as important for finding balance in work and life.

- Participants were concerned about their ability to focus on patients.

- Competing demands in the work environment became a barrier to focusing on patients' agendas.

Ferrell (2006) examined nurses' moral distress in 108 narratives about end-of-life care experiences; the narratives were written by nurses who attended continuing education courses. The most common experience contributing to nurses' moral distress was continuing aggressive, futile care that overshadowed the benefits of palliative care. In addition, nurses identified moral distress that resulted from conflicts with physicians, patients, and family members.

Stressors Encountered in Caring for Patients and Families at the End of Life

Workload Pressures
- Staff shortages.
- Poor cooperation or accessibility of other health professionals.
- Unsupportive work environment.
- Lack of resources, including time, for meeting job expectations.
- Lack of appreciation for nurses' efforts.
- Frequent phone calls from family members wanting updates.
- Inadequate preparation for responding to end-of-life care situations.
- Gap between idealistic goals and reality of the situation.

Relationships With Other Health Professionals
- Physicians' unwillingness to listen to nurses, discuss symptom control, or trust nurses' judgment.
- Not having the same priorities as other interdisciplinary team members and allied health professionals.
- Conflict with care versus cure philosophies.
- Professional isolation, feeling invisible.
- Lack of rewards, such as recognition for contributions.

Causes of Sadness Concerning Care Situations
- Over-identification with patients and families.
- Working with younger patients.
- Working with family members who do not accept a patient's death.

- Lack of control over symptom relief or other difficult situations.
- Conflict with family members.
- A long and painful dying process.
- Continuing aggressive and futile care.
- Confronting issues of own mortality.
- Accumulation of sadness from numerous deaths.

Sources: Ablett & Jones, 2007; Badger, 2005; Barnes, 2001; Ferrell, 2006; Jenull & Brunner, 2008; Lambert & Lambert, 2008; Newton & Walters, 2001; Rose & Glass, 2006; Sabo, 2008; Vachon, 2006; Zerwekh, 2006

Health care staff who have not learned about and embraced a palliative care philosophy may perceive death as contributing to their burden. In an Austrian study of nursing home employees from a variety of disciplines, participants described situations that contributed to their burden, such as the sudden and unexpected death of residents, their emotional involvement with patients, long and difficult dying processes, and family members who were difficult to handle because they did not accept the resident's death (Jenull & Brunner, 2008).

In the intensive care setting, Beckstrand and Kirchhoff (2005) measured the intensity and frequency of obstacles experienced by intensive care nurses ($n = 1,049$) in their efforts to provide high quality end-of-life care. Obstacles in the care environment that prevent nurses from providing high quality end-of-life care contribute to their experience of stress. Nurses rated physician and family behaviors among the highest in obstacle intensity and frequency. Highest rated obstacles included multiple physicians with differing opinions about goals of care, frequent phone calls from family members who wanted updates, and physicians who avoided direct conversation with patients and families about prognosis. Another obstacle that nurses rated high in intensity was family members not understanding the effects of lifesaving measures on patients.

What Happens When Stress Is Not Managed

If nurses do not manage the stressors that are inherent in their end-of-life care, compassion fatigue or burnout may lead to ineffectiveness or contribute to their own harm or that of others in their nursing practice. The stress may carry over to their life outside of work. Helping professionals may experience compassion fatigue when they become preoccupied with another's suffering. Risk for compassion fatigue is increased in work environments that are noncollaborative and lack social support (Babant, 2001; Sabo, 2008). Burnout is a feeling connected with work that is mentally or physically exhausting. Although nurses are committed to their work, organizational factors and the mismatch between personal characteristics and abilities and expectations for job performance contribute to ongoing stress that leads to exhaustion (Babant; Sabo).

Consequences of Unmanaged Stress

- Decreased job satisfaction.

- Increased absence from work.

- Lower quality of care.

- Difficulty separating private life from work life.

- Maladaptive coping strategies, such as spending less time with dying patients.

- A sense of failure.

- Inability to concentrate and poor clinical judgment.

- Physical symptoms such as headaches and insomnia.

- Poor eating and sleeping habits, substance abuse, and procrastination.

- Perception of patients as objects and focus on high-tech aspects of end-of-life care.

- Feelings of powerlessness, helplessness, and hopelessness.

- Interdisciplinary power struggles.

Sources: Barnes, 2001; Jenull & Brunner, 2008; Jezuit, 1988; Lambert & Lambert, 2008; Mariano, 2006; Sabo, 2008; Sherman, 2006; Zerwekh, 2006

How Nurses Cope With the Challenges of End-of-Life Care

Nurses cope with the challenging demands of end-of-life care by changing their behaviors and perceptions in an effort to manage the demands (Lambert & Lambert, 2008). Coping strategies can be adaptive or maladaptive and can be focused on solving the problem or managing emotions (Payne, 2001). A problem-focused coping strategy involves taking action to change the situation or to initiate self care. An emotion-focused coping strategy involves creating a meaning that reframes the situation in a positive way. Action is intended to foster personal growth.

In a review of literature on managing emotion in palliative care nursing with children, Maunder (2008) discussed the concept of emotional labor. Emotional labor in public service roles involves managing the feelings and emotions that result from caring and interacting with others. For example, the emotional labor of nurses who provide care to terminally ill children is intense, because of the challenges of maintaining professional boundaries while providing family-centered care, addressing developmental needs of children, and sometimes being involved with a family for a long period. Nurses manage their emotions by maintaining a neutrality or distance from the emotional demands of work, or by developing an awareness that helps them understand how to manage emotions.

Froggatt (1998) found that hospice nurses "switched on and off" to avoid burnout. When emotions are too intense, nurses may avoid becoming emotionally attached to a patient and family. The nurse may focus on tasks, which decreases emotional involvement or identification with a patient and family. However, Benner and Wrubel (1989) suggested that if a nurse works too hard to not become involved, stress may result from the emotional effort needed to maintain distance. By focusing on becoming aware as opposed to distancing, nurses work to understand what is important to a child and family and can then provide the care that makes sense to that child and family. The developing awareness approach creates shared meaning with patients and families and greater satisfaction for nurses (Maunder, 2008).

A Swedish study indicated how health team members (a mix of professions, including nurses) responded to difficult situations in caring for patients with advanced cancer. The health team members balanced closeness and distance as they worked with families (Blomberg & Sahlberg-Blom, 2007). Participants described using self as a tool in daily interactions and viewing their work as important and meaningful. Limit setting kept team members from too much involvement or becoming too close to patients and families. Touching, both physically and in the spiritual sense, facilitated closeness and reciprocal relationships among staff members, patients, and families. Participants explained that they distanced patients by prioritizing the completion of routine duties or focusing on symptoms that could be easily managed. Colleagues that complemented and strengthened each other facilitated closeness, while a hierarchical team approach resulted in distancing. Participants believed the palliative care philosophy resulted in greater closeness in comparison to traditional care.

"Finding meaning and purpose in your work can counteract the negative consequences of stress."

In a study of medical intensive care nurses who cared for patients being transitioned to comfort care, Badger (2005) found the nurses used cognitive, affective, and behavioral coping strategies:

* *Cognitive Strategies*—putting up with knowing that death was coming, visualizing the patient as a family member to promote empathy, learning from experience, remembering past patient experiences, and putting things into perspective by not taking the situation home.

* *Affective Strategies*—using humor to reduce tensions, externalizing feelings by verbalizing frustrations, and emotionally compartmentalizing by separating self from work events and not talking about what people do not want to hear.

* *Behavioral Strategies*—retreating from a patient care assignment by walking away or being dismissed from the assignment, and distancing self from difficult families.

In addition, personal factors affect coping responses, including an awareness of what contributes to nurses' perceptions of stress and faith or religious beliefs (Barnes, 2001).

Taking Charge of Self-Care

We experience many rewards in our work with patients and families in end-of-life care. As nurses, we interact with patients and families, acknowledge the importance of life, and help patients and families to find meaning in their end-of-life experiences. Finding meaning and purpose in your work can counteract the negative consequences of stress. Studies have found that palliative care staff members have lower levels of burnout in comparison with other specialties (Vachon, 2006). We can also strengthen our resilience in dealing with stress by taking action to promote physical, emotional, spiritual, and social health. Resilience is not about avoiding stress. Rather, resilience develops as people respond to or manage stress in ways that increase self-confidence, social competence, and mastery of responsibilities (Rutter, 1985).

In interviews with 10 English hospice nurses, Ablett and Jones (2007) explored factors that promote resilience. The resulting themes reflected nurses' perceptions about having a high level of commitment and sense of purpose in their work. The nurses had chosen to work in palliative care and were committed to making a difference in their role. Their work led to an awareness of their own mortality and a zest for living. They identified a need to have manageable tasks and a sense of control over their work. Receiving social support and sharing work with colleagues contributed to their work satisfaction. They also recognized the need for humor, a healthy work-life balance, and maintaining an awareness of their professional boundaries (a protective factor).

Only in taking care of ourselves can we make a positive difference in the lives of patients and families who are on an end-of-life journey. Babant (2001) suggested the following rules nurses can use to keep self-care responsibilities in perspective:

- It is my responsibility to take care of myself.

- It is my responsibility to find the kind of self-care that is best suited to my particular needs.

- It is important to see myself as part of a larger process; it is also important to see myself as a unique and important part of that process and thus, deserving of self-care.

- Only then can I be of help and comfort to others (p. 452).

"Only in taking care of ourselves can we make a positive difference in the lives of patients and families who are on an end-of-life-journey."

Maslow's hierarchy can be used as a framework to identify self-care strategies. Starting with the base of the hierarchical triangle, self-care strategies suggested by Zerwekh (2006) include:

1. Focus on breathing.

2. Develop healthy eating patterns.

3. Create an exercise plan that is feasible.

4. Exercise the mind by reducing self-criticism and creating a positive self-message.

5. Surround yourself with a caring community and social network.

6. Exercise your spirit through worship, prayer, renewal in art and music, and meditation.

Self-Care Strategies for Nurses Who Provide End-of-Life Care

Perceptual Strategies

- Identify the stressors that affect your well-being in the workplace (Rose & Glass, 2006).

- Take responsibility for your stress and know your own limitations; identify coping mechanisms that can help you manage the stress effectively (Barnes, 2001).

- Reduce unnecessary stress by saying "no," removing yourself from stress-producing people when possible, avoiding controversial topics if not essential to work, and shortening your "to do" list (Lambert & Lambert, 2008).

- Change perceptions about the stressor—express feelings, reframe the problem, define the big picture, adjust standards, look for the positive (Lambert & Lambert, 2008).

- Accept what you cannot change—let go of the desire to control; forgive others (Lambert & Lambert, 2008).

- Reflect on the rewards of giving end-of-life care and the contributions that you have made to the lives of patients and families (Sherman, 2006).

- Take time to reflect on experiencing patients' deaths and the lessons that you can learn from the experience (Sherman, 2006).

- Talk with colleagues or keep a journal about feelings and perceptions (Sherman, 2006).

Maintaining a Healthy Work/Life Balance

- Use appropriate humor to relieve tension (Ablett & Jones, 2007).

- Cultivate your social support network (Ablett & Jones, 2007).

- Take care of your spiritual needs (Touhy & Zerwekh, 2006).
  - Participate in your faith traditions.
  - Take time for reflection and meditation.
  - Spend time with nature and the arts.

- Take care of personal needs (Lambert & Lambert, 2008).
  - Schedule time for relaxation.

- Do something enjoyable every day.
- Exercise regularly.
- Eat nutritious foods.
- Avoid substance abuse.

- Make a list of life goals and a plan for working on what you would like to accomplish (Babant 2001) that includes:

  - Social support (consider looking outside of work and family).
  - Personal physical care, including adequate rest.
  - Ways to mange emotions.
  - Intellectual development (nursing profession and beyond).
  - Spiritual growth for connectedness to God and others.

- Share your plan with a support person to encourage accountability (Henry & Henry, 2004).

What Organization Leaders Can Do to Promote Self-Care

Leaders of health care organizations can create an environment that helps nurses integrate self-care approaches into their work. This can be done through supporting effective teamwork, promoting interdisciplinary collaboration, and offering educational programs.

Supporting Teamwork

By creating processes and setting aside time for team development, members of the team can recognize the various skills that complement their own expertise and strengths. Effective team interactions can help each member more effectively manage the emotional labor encountered in their work (Maunder, 2008). Expert members of the team can offer clinical supervision, mentoring, and peer support to novices (Newton & Waters, 2001; Caton & Klemm, 2006). Leaders in health care organizations at all levels—hospitals, long-term care and assisted-living facilities, hospices, and home care—should structure regular opportunities for dialogue. In providing these opportunities to talk, leaders show respect for the team, which helps build trusting and caring relationships (Vachon, 2006). In addition, organizational leaders should pay attention to the workload of staff members and the impact on patient care, as well as provide a process for debriefing and reflection in difficult situations (Grbich et al., 2006).

Improving Interdisciplinary Collaboration

Bronstein (2003) offers a conceptual framework with core components that contribute to successful collaboration for interdisciplinary teams.

- Interdependence.

- Newly created professional activities—programs, structures, collaborative actions that would not be possible independently.

- Flexibility.

- Collective ownership of goals.

- Reflection on the process.

Synergy, in which more is accomplished than one person alone can accomplish, results from collaboration. Collaboration in which professionals learn to rely on knowledge and interactions with other disciplines contributes to better communication.

Using Bronstein's model, Oliver and Peck (2006) explored social workers' perspectives of their experience with hospice team collaboration. They identified the following strategies for improving interdisciplinary collaboration in the hospice setting:

- Conduct joint visits with colleagues from different disciplines.

- Participate in team-building activities.

- Respect other team members' roles, allowing for some "blurring" of roles in the hospice setting.

- Obtain administrative support for time and resources for team building and external networking on best practices in hospice.

Educational Strategies

Educating disciplines together about the precepts of palliative care and effective strategies is another strategy for improving interdisciplinary communication (Egan & Abbott, 2002; Koffman, 2001). Content should be presented at a level understandable to all participants. Equitable participation in interdisciplinary communication can help all participants recognize their skill sets and overcome biases concerning other professions.

Canadian researchers created a psycho-educational group intervention to create meaning-making opportunities to reduce the stress encountered in palliative care nursing (Fillion, Dupuis, Tremblay, de Grace, & Breitbart, 2006). The group intervention for professionals included four weekly meetings that addressed characteristics and sources of meaning; personal values and a sense of accomplishment at work; and meaning encountered in suffering, humor, and emotional experiences. Educational methods included a handbook with didactic presentation handouts, home exercises, and the book *Tuesdays with Morrie*, which is about emotional connection with a dying man. Following completion of the four sessions, nurses were asked to write short essays about meaningful experiences in their palliative care nurse practice, which offered a way to share their learning and experiences with others.

Narratives of end-of-life care offer a teaching tool for managing the emotional stress related to working with dying patients. In an analysis of 105 published narratives of professionals in end-of-life care settings, researchers found the stories showed how to manage the emotional tensions present in these settings (Wittenberg-Lyles, Greene, & Sanchez-Reilly, 2007). Such narratives explain the attitudes and approaches to end-of-life care that prepare practitioners to respond effectively to challenges without succumbing to the stress of difficult situations.

Sherman (2006) poses questions that educators can ask to help nurses and nursing students develop awareness of their own self-care needs and identify ways to achieve their well-being:

* What expectations do you have about yourself in caring for the dying and bereaved?

- What would define success in your work?

- What are the three most difficult aspects of your work in caring for patients with life-threatening illness?

- What are you doing to help yourself cope with stress and replenish your energy to avoid becoming overstressed? (p. 32)

Reflective Practice

Emphasizing the rewards of end-of-life care helps frame the positive experiences of what we do. However, even positive experiences become diminished with over-work and a sense of being overwhelmed. At these times, we need to communicate with our inner selves by reflecting about what is happening and taking action to stop the spiral of stress. We need to develop our own self-care strategies and a support system to help cushion the sharp edges of our work to prevent "hard landings" that could bring about illness or the desire to leave a job.

The virtues of humility, self-confidence, honesty, and courage can help us real-ize that we need and benefit from the support of others as we work to help our patients and families navigate their end-of-life journey. In humility, we recognize what we have to offer in end-of-life care and value the expertise and contributions of our health care team members. With self-confidence, we can move forward with self-care strategies that contribute to the health of our own body, mind, and spirit. In our wholeness, we will have the ability to do our best work. In situations of overload, we need honesty to diagnose our own developing stress spiral and have the courage to take action to stop the spiral.

Ethical Practice in Promoting Self-Care

ETHICAL PROBLEM: As a supervisor, how should I respond to hospice home care nurses who have been taking an increasing number of sick days, which has negative consequences for the quality of care provided?

What Should I Value?

- Quality end-of-life care for patients enrolled in hospice.

- A satisfying work experience for nurses.

- Retention of competent nurses.

Who Should I Be?

- An honest and courageous supervisor who is willing to communicate concern and take needed action.

- A nurse who respects the perceptions of those nurses.

- A nurse who has self-confidence in the process of gathering evidence about the problem and identifying strategies to respond appropriately.

What Should I Do?

- Collect data about nurses' perceptions of what is contributing to increasing sick days.

- Evaluate the fairness of the workload.

- Strategize about ways to accomplish work more efficiently (e.g., reconfigure assignments based on geographic area, introduce new technology).

- Meet with interdisciplinary team members to brainstorm about alternative structures for delivering care.

- Offer a monthly meeting for support and a debriefing opportunity (could be led by a chaplain or social worker).

- Seek outside consultation if chosen actions do not result in improvement.

Let go, do something new, take a break, know that others care—these are actions that you can take when you are feeling overwhelmed by the many demands and expectations encountered in your work. When you balance the demands of work with self-care strategies, you will experience the satisfaction of knowing that what you do makes a difference not only to you but also to your patients, their families, and your co-workers.

Nurses' Stories

Rewards in End-of-Life Care

One of the best ways to avoid compassion fatigue is to look at the rewards in caring for dying patients. A Norwegian nurse working in a nursing home describes her experience:

> We have a routine after people have passed away. We always clean the room and take away books and papers and equipment—everything. We freshen [the deceased] up a bit and put them on a white cloth on the table. We lay the Bible there, and then the family can go in. And they can be with us when we are taking care of them afterwards if they want to. A woman's husband asked me about what I was doing. I told him everything I did. He came to me after the funeral and said thank you.

The same nurse spoke about another family:

> I went to the funeral. The daughter came afterwards and thanked me for good care and gave us flowers—lovely. And then you know you have done a good job. She was one of my primary patients. That was special.

Sometimes rewards do not come from a thank-you or compliment, but from the satisfaction of knowing that our work makes a difference in the well-being of patients and families. The following story from a Norwegian nurse illustrates that it is important for family members to have a sense of peace in their own journey with the dying person. In this reflection, the nurse knows the young boy will have a good memory of his relationship with his grandfather. It is an experience that makes the nurse's work worthwhile.

It's about the grandfather and his grandson. The grandfather was a de-pressed man. He was just wanting to die. After having a discussion with his wife, daughter, and grandson, I realized that the grandson had been really close to his grandfather. When the boy visited his grandfather though, the boy would just cry all the time. It was difficult for the grandfather. He complained and one time said, "Oh, just take that kid home." It sounded like he didn't want his grandson there. He sounded angry. After I talked to the family, I realized that it didn't have to be like that. So, before the wife and family came back in, I talked to him about the grandson. I said, "He's just a teenager," and I told him that it was difficult for the boy, that he needed to be there-even though he cried, he had to be there. The grand-father didn't respond to me, but when the boy came back into the room again, the grandfather opened his arms and said, "come here and sit by my side. I have to tell you how I love you so." They had had so much together-fishing, mountains-and this gesture from the grandfather helped the boy be okay with his coming loss. We cried, watching them. And later that day it was a much easier atmosphere in the room. When the boy left that day, he said "love you, Grandpa. Come back soon." And that's the way they had talked before. I think it helped this boy for the rest of his life. He is going to live on. He was able to share with his grandfather what he felt.

Self-Care

A hospice nurse writes about journaling as a means of self-care.

I have found great value in writing stories and rereading them. When I find myself caught up in the sadness of patient losses, I sit with these sto-ries, experiencing my connections to the patients over and over again. This is what I advise to others about journaling:

- *Write from where you are.*
- *Try writing a conversation with a patient.*
- *Write what you miss about patients.*
- *Write what you've learned from patients.*
- *Write about how knowing patients and being part of their dying have affected your life.*

Nurses spend so much time caring for others that they don't always take the time to care for themselves. A hospice nurse relates how she's "carved out" time for herself:

> Every two weeks I have my nails done. I've been going to the same manicurist for the last 10 years. It's the one regular time in my life when someone else takes care of me. It's sacred time for me, and I hardly ever miss my appointments.

Support Within Organizations

A long-term care nurse described support for the staff within her facility:

> When a patient dies, we have a memorial service for both the staff and the residents. It feels good to honor the patients who have passed, and it's a chance for everyone to tell stories about those patients.

On the other hand, an ICU nurse noted that part of the stress in having a patient die was the inability to talk about it:

> I need to talk about that patient and to tell the story, but on our unit, we are so busy we simply move on. Sometimes it makes it hard to come back the next day.

Key Points

To be present for patients and families, nurses need to recognize stressors and practice self-care.

- Common stressors include workload pressures, relationships with other health care professionals, and grief and sadness related to the dying and loss of patients.

- Unmanaged stress can result in physical and mental exhaustion, dissatisfaction with the job, lower quality of care, and feelings of sadness and powerlessness.

- Coping with stress includes using the interdisciplinary team for support, setting limits, and finding meaning in work.

- Self-care includes having healthy eating and exercise patterns, surrounding yourself with a supportive community, taking the time to reflect on the rewards of your work, and developing a work-life balance.

REFLECTION QUESTIONS

1. What situations in end-of-life care have been emotionally challenging for you? What did you do to manage your emotions?

2. Think about someone you know who is resilient in the presence of stress. What do you think has contributed to his or her resilience?

3. Develop a self-care plan that includes specific strategies for personal physical care, management of emotions, social support, intellectual development, and spiritual growth.

References

Ablett, J. R., & Jones, R. S. P. (2007). Resilience and well-being in palliative care staff: A qualitative study of hospice nurses' experience of work. *Psycho-Oncology, 16*, 733-740.

Babant, S. (2001). Taking care of yourself. In B. Poor & G. P. Poirrier, (Eds.), *End of life nursing care* (pp. 443-453). Sudbury, MA: Jones and Bartlett.

Badger, J. M. (2005). A descriptive study of coping strategies used by medical intensive care unit nurses during transitions from cure- to comfort-oriented care. *Heart & Lung, 34*(10), 63-68.

Barnes, K. (2001). Staff stress in the children's hospice: Causes, effects and coping strategies. *International Journal of Palliative Nursing, 7*(5), 248-254.

Benner, P., & Wrubel, J. (1989). *The primacy of caring.* Menlo Park, CA: Addison-Wesley.

Blomberg, K., & Sahlberg-Blom, E. (2007). Closeness and distance: A way of handling difficult situations in daily care. *Journal of Clinical Nursing, 16*, 244-254.

Bronstein, L. R. (2003). A model for interdisciplinary collaboration. *Social Work, 48*(3), 297-306.

Bruce, A. (2008). The changing landscape of palliative care: Emotional challenges for hospice palliative care professionals. *Journal of Hospice & Palliative Nursing, 10*(1), 49-55.

Caton, A. P., & Klemm, P. (2006). Introduction of novice oncology nurses to end-of-life care. *Clinical Journal of Oncology Nursing, 10*(5), 604-608.

Egan, K. A., & Abbott, P. (2002). Interdisciplinary team training: Preparing nurse employees for the specialty of hospice and palliative care. *Journal of Hospice and Palliative Nursing, 4*(3), 161-171.

Ferrell, B. R. (2006). Understanding the moral distress of nurses witnessing medically futile care. *Oncology Nursing Forum, 33*(5), 922-930.

Fillion, L., Dupuis, R., Tremblay, I., de Grace, G., & Breitbart, W. (2006). Enhancing meaning in palliative care practice: A meaning-centered intervention to promote job satisfaction. *Palliative and Supportive Care, 4*, 333-344.

Froggatt, K. (1998). The place of metaphor and language in exploring nurses' emotional work. *Journal of Advanced Nursing, 28*, 332-338.

Grbich, C., Parish, K., Glaetzer, K., Hegarty, M., Hammond, L., & McHugh, A. (2006). Communication and decision making for patients with end stage diseases in an acute care setting. *Contemporary Nurse, 23*, 21-37.

Henry, L. G., & Henry, J. D. (2004). *The soul of the caring nurse: Stories and resources for revitalizing professional passion.* Washington, DC: American Nurses Association.

Jenull, B., & Brunner, E. (2008). Death and dying in nursing homes: A burden for the staff? *Journal of Applied Gerontology, 27*(2), 166-180.

Jezuit, D. L. (1988). The phases of suffering experienced by critical care nurses in association with difficult end-of-life situations. UMI Dissertation Services. (UMI No. 3000501).

Koffman, J. (2001). Multiprofessional palliative care education: Past challenges, future issues. *Journal of Palliative Care, 17*(2), 86-92.

Lambert, V. A., & Lambert, C. E. (2008). Nurses' workplace stressors and coping strategies. *Indian Journal of Palliative Care, 14*(1), 38-44.

Mariano, C. (2006). Holistic integrative therapies. In M. L. Matzo & D. W. Sherman (Eds.), *Palliative care nursing: Quality care to the end of life* (pp. 51-86). New York: Springer.

Maunder, E. Z. (2008). Emotion management in children's palliative care nursing. *Indian Journal of Palliative Care, 14*(1), 45-50.

Newton, J., & Waters, V. (2001). Community palliative care clinical nurse specialists' descriptions of stress in their work. *International Journal of Palliative Nursing, 7*(11), 531-540.

Oliver, D. P., & Peck, M. (2006). Inside the interdisciplinary team experiences of hospice social workers. *Journal of Social Work in End-of-Life & Palliative Care, 2*(3), 7-21.

Payne, N. (2001). Occupational stressors and coping as determinants of burnout in female hospice nurses. *Journal of Advanced Nursing, 33*, 396-405.

Rose, J., & Glass, N. (2006). Nurses and palliation in the community: The current discourse. *International Journal of Palliative Nursing, 12*(12), 588-594.

Rutter, M. (1985). Resilience in the face of adversity: Protective factors and resistance to psychiatric disorder. *The British Journal of Psychiatry, 147*, 598-611.

Sabo, B. M. (2008). Adverse psychosocial consequences: Compassion fatigue, burnout and vicarious traumatization: Are nurses who provide palliative and hematological cancer care vulnerable? *Indian Journal of Palliative Care, 14*(1), 23-29.

Sherman, D. W. (2006). Spirituality and culture as domains of quality palliative care. In M. L. Matzo & D. W. Sherman (Eds.), *Palliative care nursing: Quality care to the end of life* (pp. 3-49). New York: Springer.

Touhy, T., & Zwerekh, J. (2006). Spiritual caring. In J. V. Zerwekh, *Nursing care at the end of life* (pp. 213-239). Philadelphia: F. A. Davis.

Vachon, M. L. S. (2006). The experience of the nurse in end-of-life care in the 21st century. In B. R. Ferrell & N. Coyle (Eds.), *Textbook of palliative nursing* (pp. 1011-1029). New York: Oxford University Press.

Wittenberg-Lyles, E. M., Greene, K., & Sanchez-Reilly, S. (2007). Using published narratives as a teaching tool in end-of-life care. *Journal of Hospice and Palliative Nursing, 9*(4), 198-205.

Zerwekh, J. (2006). *Nursing care at the end of life.* Philadelphia: F. A. Davis.

A

•

The Nurses' Stories

The nurses' stories represent experiences of expert nurses from the United States and Norway. The inspiration for the book and the themes of the chapters originate from Marjorie Schaffer's travel to Norway in 2005 for the Fulbright Scholar Program. Schaffer selected Norway as a site for the end-of-life research to explore ethical problems in end-of-life care in a country with universal health care; in addition, her own Scandinavian heritage influenced her decision to focus on Norway. Over a 4-month stay, Schaffer (2007) interviewed 25 Norwegian health professionals, 6 elders, and 5 family members about the ethical problems they experienced in end-of-life decision-making in Norway. Seventeen nurses participated in the study; they worked in a variety of health care settings in Norway, and all had extensive experience in providing end-of-life care. The research focused on end-of-life care for elders.

Norwegian health professionals experienced the following kinds of ethical problems:

1. Difficult relationships with family members.

2. Concern about the quality of health care services.

3. Disagreement among health professionals.

4. Problematic treatment decisions.

5. Not knowing how to involve elders in decision-making.

6. Overcoming a reluctance to discuss death and dying.

7. Managing own feelings and burdens of providing care.

8. Knowing how to meet spiritual needs.

Beyond the analysis for expression of ethical problems, the nurses' stories provided rich narratives about the meaning of their work—the challenges and rewards they encountered in giving end-of-life care. Many of these stories were about communication—what worked well, what did not, how to begin conversations about dying, and how to respond to people who were not ready to talk. A number of their stories are found throughout this book. The stories reveal important values that nurses hold in caring for patients at the end of life, the kind of nurse they wish to be in their work, and their challenges and struggles in deciding how to best deliver quality end-of-life care.

The Norwegian nurses' stories suggested communication themes that describe strategies and challenges as nurses communicate with patients, families, and interdisciplinary staff about end-of-life care situations. To expand the pool of stories, Linda Norlander invited expert nurses who had extensive experience in end-of-life care to participate in a focus group to discuss their work. Norlander and Schaffer used the themes suggested by the Norwegian study to frame statements and questions for additional exploration of communication themes:

1. Share your thoughts on what it means to be present with patients and families. Describe a time when you believed your presence and what you did made a difference for them.

2. How do you know what to say to patients and families about dying? Give some examples of when you knew it was the right time to talk with them about dying and preparing for death.

3. Tell us how you respond to wishes and hopes expressed by patients and families. Give an example of a time when you had to respond to unreasonable or impossible wishes. What did you say? How did they respond?

4. Describe a situation where you talked with a patient/family about the spiritual aspect of dying.

5. Describe a time when you had to deal with significant conflict with a patient or family. What helped you?

6. Tell us about a situation where you misunderstood what a patient or family wanted or needed. What did you do?

7. Share your thoughts and examples of times when you needed to take action for the safety of the patient or family.

8. How do you say good-bye to your patients and families? How do you guide them in saying good-bye?

9. Describe examples of working with patients and families of different cultural and ethnic backgrounds. What conflicts did you encounter? What lessons did you learn?

10. How do you promote advance care planning in your practice and also in your personal life?

Five nurses participated in the focus group. All had experience working with patients at the end of life in a variety of settings, including hospice, home care, children's home care, intensive care, and long-term care. The group included an ICU nurse, clinical nurse specialist in palliative care and a geriatric nurse practitioner, as well as two nurses certified in hospice and palliative care. The focus group data were transcribed and analyzed by grouping quotes for each question theme. A number of these stories were selected to illustrate key meanings and experiences that were especially relevant to the chapter topics.

A third source of stories was from the professional work of Norlander, who has ongoing dialogues with hospice and palliative care nurses. She has written two books on end-of-life care: *To Comfort Always: A Nurse's Guide to End of Life Care* (2008) and *Choices at the End of Life: Finding Out What Your Parents Want Before It's Too Late* (2001, with Kerstin McSteen). In addition, she has published in numerous professional journals on advance care planning, communication, and suffering at the end of life. Her long-standing relationships with nurses in practice have brought her stories that represent the everyday practice of nurses who care for patients at the end of life. As a manager of a home care and hospice organization, Norlander navigates the challenges of the health care system with nurses to reach the goal of providing quality care to dying patients and their family members.

Reference

Schaffer, M. A. (2007). Ethical problems in end-of-life decisions for elderly Norwegians. *Nursing Ethics, 14*(2), 243-257.

Additional Reading

Norlander, L. (2008). *To comfort always: A nurse's guide to end-of-life care*. Indianapolis, IN: Sigma Theta Tau International.

Norlander, L., & McSteen, K. (2001). *Choices at the end of life: Finding out what your parents want before it's too late*. Minneapolis, MN: Fairview Press.

B

•

The Checklist of Family Relational Abilities

Check the descriptions below (one for each category) that best describe the family you are working with. The term "family member" is used to include the patient as well as any other involved individual who has biological, legal, or emotional ties to the patient.

Attachment Bonds

_____ Strong, positive bonds of affection are apparent among all or nearly all family members.

_____ Attachment bonds appear to be weak, ambivalent, or "mixed" (i.e., both positive bonds and conflictual relationships in the family).

_____ Intense conflict or "wounded" relationships are apparent among most or all family members.

Openness of Communication Regarding the Current Illness

_____ Communication among all or nearly all family members is open and includes expression of emotional reactions to the illness.

_____ Most family members discuss the illness openly, but some individuals are excluded and/or avoid expression of emotional reactions.

_____ Some family members discuss the facts of the illness, but few family members are involved in the discussions and/or emotional reactions are not shared.

_____ There is little if any discussion of the illness among family members.

Collaborative Decision-Making Regarding the Current Illness

_____ Most or all family members participate in decision-making, and most seem satisfied with decisions that are made.

_____ Decisions are made by a minority of family members (e.g., the patient alone or one or two family members), but others accept or have grown to accept the decisions.

_____ Decisions are made by a minority of family members, causing others to feel left out and unsatisfied with the decisions on an ongoing basis.

_____ The family has great difficulty making decisions and/or there is serious, ongoing conflict about decisions that are made.

Overall Level of Family Relational Abilities

Circle the number below that best describes the overall capabilities and needs of the family you are working with:

4. **Naturally Resilient:** Predominately strong, positive bonds of attachment; clear and open communication; effective, collaborative decision-making (little if any family intervention needed)

3. **Overwhelmed:** Predominately strong relational abilities but temporarily stymied by intensity and/or complexity of the patient's situation (brief family support may help engage natural abilities)

2. **Closed or Fixed:** Significant difficulties with communication and/or decision-making (targeted intervention or family consultation may help open communication and/or facilitate decision-making)

1. **Wounded:** Damaged bonds of attachment, intensely negative or conflictual communication and/or decision making (family therapy indicated to address longstanding grievances among family members)

Comments:

Source: Wilkins, V. M., King, D. A., & Quill, T. E. (In Press). Assessing families in palliative care: A pilot study of the Checklist of Family Relational Abilities. Journal of Palliative Medicine.

Index

A

Q-R